Praise for *Your Dog's Golden Years*

Your Dog's Golden Years, edited by Jennifer Kachnic, CCMT, CRP, fills a long-standing need for owners of elderly canines. Chapters are written by specialists in various aspects of canine care.

The book is thorough, starting with the basics: benefits of adopting a senior dog, senior nutrition, supplements useful for seniors, bloodwork and other basic information with an emphasis on the senior dog, and dental care. A chapter describes how older dogs think and feel, which is very different from young puppies.

In addition, it addresses the special problems of seniors, including common medical conditions, with a discussion of what can be done for them. As chronic diseases these are often very responsive to complementary techniques such as acupuncture, chiropractic, herbs, aromatherapy, and physical therapy. There is a chapter on each one of these modalities.

And finally, there is a discussion of end-of-life issues. Hospice care and euthanasia are discussed, as well as a chapter on dealing with your own feelings after an older pet's death.

Your Dog's Golden Years is ideal for anyone owning a dog: sooner or later your dog will be in the senior category, and this reference covers major categories that you will need to know.

Dr. Nancy Scanlan, Executive Director,
American Holistic Veterinary Medical Association

Your Dog's Golden Years is an essential read not just for anyone who owns a senior or geriatric dog, but anyone who owns a dog. It is a wonderful blend of traditional and complementary care for dogs, with an eloquent explanation of the science and rationale behind many tests and treatments for aging dogs. Often times pet caregivers experience an 'information overload' when their pet is diagnosed with a life-threatening or terminal illness. 'Golden Years' is the perfect reference to explain

D0054988

and inform caregivers of what their dog may be experiencing in the present or near future. This book should be in the waiting room of all veterinary practices!

Marti Drum DVM, PhD, CCRP, CERP
Clinical Assistant Professor, Small Animal Physical Rehabilitation,
University of Tennessee, Veterinary Teaching Hospital

Your Dog's Golden Years, edited by Jennifer Kachnic, CCMT, CRP, fills a long-standing need for owners of elderly canines. Chapters are written by specialists in various aspects of canine care.

Your Dog's Golden Years is a well written, thoughtful and comprehensive guide to taking care of your furry friends as they age.

This outstanding book will help dog parents ensure that their companion is happy and as comfortable as possible through their senior years. Kudos to Jennifer Kachnic and the other authors for compiling such a complete resource guide for dog parent's everywhere. A must read.

Jennifer Brauns, Publisher of *Mile High Dog Magazine*

Dogs get better as they get older, but like their human companions, they slow with age – and then they leave us all too soon. Jennifer Kachnic and the 19 other experts in this book offer hundreds of solutions for dozens of problems that affect older dogs. With up-to-date treatments like lasers, ancient and modern remedies from medicinal plants, laboratory test guidelines for elderly patients, hands-on healing techniques, "old dog" training tips, senior nutrition, strategies for dealing with end-of-life decisions, and helpful advice for caregivers, *Your Dog's Golden Years* is truly comprehensive. No matter how much you know about canine health and behavior, you'll learn something important and your best friend will benefit for years to come.

CJ Puotinen, author of *The Encyclopedia of Natural Pet Care*
and *Natural Remedies for Dogs and Cats*

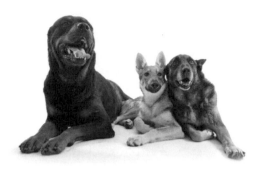

Contributing Authors

Claude, Senior Dog Spokesman
Canine Wellness, Denver, Colorado

Sherri Franklin & Liz Brooking
Muttville Senior Dog Rescue – San Francisco, California

Brian Lapham, DVM, CVA
Southpoint Veterinary Clinic – Durham, North Carolina

Terri O'Hara
Animalwize Animal Communication – Corvallis, Oregon

Susan Lauten, PhD
Pet Nutrition Consulting – Knoxville, Tennessee

Fred Metzger, DVM Diplomate, ABVP
Metzger Animal Hospital – State College, Pennsylvania

Maia Bazjanac, CADH
Pettooth Dental Cleaning – Oakland, California

Martha Pease, CCRP, MSPT
Canine Rehabilitation & Conditioning Group –
Englewood, Colorado

Andi Harper, DC, CAC
Harper's Ridge Animal Chiropractic Care – Parker, Colorado

Erin Mayo, DVM, CVA
Vet Acupuncture – Orlando, Florida

Frances Fitzgerald Cleveland, EOS, HP
Frogworks Natural Healing – Littleton, Colorado

Brian A. Pryor, PhD, President and CEO
LiteCure Lasers – Newark, Delaware

Marcie Fallek, DVM, CVA
Holistic Vet – New York, New York

Alice Villalobos, DVM, DPNAP – Cancer Care Veterinarian
Pawspice – Woodland Hills, California

Ella Bittel, Holistic Veterinarian
Spirits in Transition – Los Alamos, California

Michelle Morrison, DVM, CVCP
Pet Home Euthanasia – Scottsdale, Arizona

Doug Koktavy, Esq.
Author – Denver, Colorado

Julie Dudley
Grey Muzzle Organization, Wake Forest, North Carolina

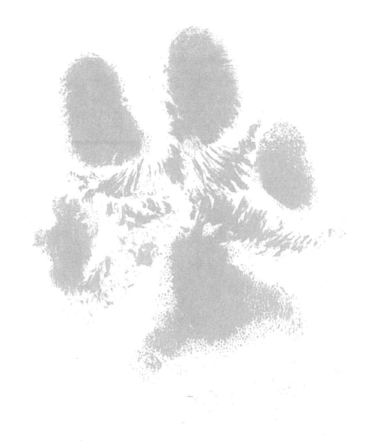

Claude's Pawtograph

Your Dog's Golden Years

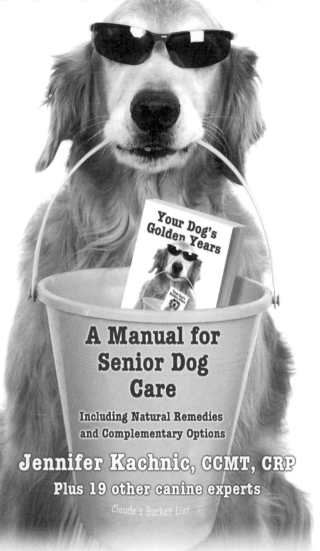

Your Dog's
Golden Years

A Manual for Senior Dog Care

Including Natural Remedies and Complementary Options

Jennifer Kachnic, CCMT, CRP

Plus 19 other canine experts

Claude's Bucket List

Your Dog's Golden Years: A Manual for Senior Dog Care
by Jennifer Kachnic
Copyright 2012 by Jennifer Kachnic

Published in the United States by Wallingford Vale Publishing
2221 E. Arapahoe Rd, #3331
Littleton, CO 80161
www.WallingfordVale.com

For more information about purchasing this book and special discounts
for bulk purchases, please contact:
Info@SeniorDogBooks.com

This book is meant to supplement the advice and guidance of your veterinarian.
No two medical conditions are the same. Moreover, we cannot be responsible for
unsupervised treatments administered at home. The techniques and suggestions are used
at the reader's discretion and are not to be considered a substitute for veterinary care.
Therefore, we urge you to search out the best medical resources available to help you
make informed decisions on your dog's care. The authors and publisher shall not be liable
in the event of incidental or consequential damages in connection with, or arising out of,
the furnishing, performance, or use of the suggestions contained in this book.

Manufactured in the United States of America
First Edition, 2012

Library of Congress
Cataloging in publication. Date is on file with the Library of Congress
1-705089150

ISBN: 978-0-9847065-1-8 (perfectbound)
ISBN: 978-0-9847065-0-1 (eBook)
Project Team
Editors: Patti Thorn, Christine Holt and Christine Gillow
Cover and Interior Designer: NZ Graphics
Book Shepherd: Judith Briles

Book Website: www.SeniorDogBooks.com

Your Dog's Golden Years is dedicated to the Grey Muzzle Organization whose goal is to enable animal welfare organizations to improve their ability to provide care, comfort, and loving homes for old dogs. The organizations that they support all have a commitment to senior dogs. They do this by raising money that is distributed annually, via grants, to animal welfare organizations and applicable rescue groups. These funds are raised through public donations; they are not a privately endowed foundation.

By providing support through grants, they help to build programs around the country that meet the special needs of senior dogs. They support only programs run by non-profit animal welfare organizations; personally evaluate each organization and program that they support; and they require accountability.

www.GreyMuzzle.org

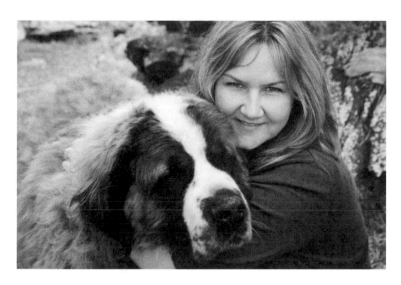

A Note from Jennifer

I would like to thank all my contributing authors for their efforts and for making this book possible. We have all dedicated our lives to providing senior dogs the care and respect they deserve.

The goal of this book is to further our mission and give you the information and tools you need to provide your senior dog with the best years yet.

I would also like to thank the following mentors, friends and family for their support:

Brianna Scroggins	John Kachnic
Christine Holt	Judith Briles
Christine Gillow	Krystal Joscelyne
Jackie Taylor	Sophia Paul
Jo Bennison	Susan Harman

Proceeds of this book will go to The Grey Muzzle Organization. www.GreyMuzzle.org

Contents

Foreword

I hope that you have been one of the lucky humans to share your life with a senior dog! If so, you have experienced the gentle joys of living together day-to-day, the amusements when your old dog suddenly dredges up a burst of insane energy from his youth, and the worries of determining the best way to care for your dog as he ages.

Your Dog's Golden Years will guide you in new ways to enjoy your moments together and improve the quality of those moments. As you delve into this book, you will feel less burdened and more excited about exploring this stage together.

I founded The Grey Muzzle Organization, a national non-profit that makes grants for senior dog care, because I learned, rather late in life, that senior dogs have much to give. They teach us about loyalty, caring, responsibility, and patience (a much-needed lesson in my case). I believe the biggest gift we can give back is to accept the responsibility, and the great rewards, of making their last years their best years.

Jennifer Kachnic has assembled an impressive group of experts for this book. I wish I could mention all of them here, but to give a sampling, you will hear from:

- Dr. Fred Metzger, a diplomat of the American Board of Veterinary Practitioners, who serves on the practitioner advisory boards of *Veterinary Economics* and *Veterinary Medicine* magazines.
- Dr. Alice Villalobos, the president of the Society for Veterinary Medical Ethics (SVME).
- Dr. Marcie Fallek, the U.S. representative to the International Academy of Veterinary Homeopathy (IAVH).

- Doug Koktavy, best-selling author of *The Legacy of Beezer and Boomer* and a certified counselor for the Association for Pet Loss and Bereavement.
- Sherri Franklin, former vice chair of the Animal Control and Welfare Commission of San Francisco, and founder and executive director of Muttville Senior Dog Rescue, which has found homes for more than 1,100 senior dogs.
- Dr. Brian Pryor, author of the book *Clinical Overview and Applications of Class IV Therapy Lasers* and founder of LiteCure, LLC, which created the Class IV laser system most used by veterinarians.
- Ella Bittel, who has specialized in holistic modalities for over 20 years, including veterinary acupuncture and chiropractic, craniosacral work, homeopathy and TTOUCH.

These and other experts will help you answer questions such as:

- What are the exact laboratory tests I should have my veterinarian do, and how often?
- How can I deal with the "anticipatory grief" I feel when I know my dog is dying?
- How can I assess the quality of life my dog is experiencing?
- How important is my dog's weight?
- What alternative or complementary treatments might be best for my dog?
- Should I consider hospice care for my dog?

A huge strength of this book is that it brings together traditional veterinarian medicine as well as alternative and complementary therapies. I find more and more people are exploring a balance of techniques to increase the quality of life for their senior dogs. Several veterinarians that I have worked with have added acupuncture and laser treatment to their practices. My own elderly dogs have benefited from canine massage and chiropractic treatment, as well as from energy healing. Hydrotherapy vastly improved the quality of life for my beloved Maxwell, whose back legs failed him at the end of his life.

Your Dog's Golden Years is about exploring new ideas. Not all of the techniques might be right for your dog, or for you. As you read, keep an open mind and listen to your instincts! Many of the tools in this book are about promoting health—but many also promote your bond with your dog. Perhaps you will be motivated to visit a canine chiropractor together, research essential oils that can augment the daily pets and rubs you give your dog or take a class on canine massage with your dog (you may be getting a cold nose nudge right now!). Perhaps you will take a more proactive role in veterinary check-ups. Perhaps you will be inspired to encourage someone else (maybe a special senior citizen in your life?) to adopt a senior dog.

If you are fortunate enough to experience the joy of sharing your life with a senior dog, this book is a true investment in your relationship.

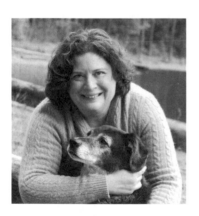

Julie Dudley
Founder of
The Grey Muzzle Organization

1

A Day in the Life of a Senior Dog with Claude

Can yawning be a sign of stress in dogs?
Do dogs handle pain differently than people?

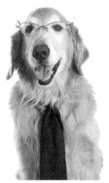

My name is Claude, and I am proud to be a 10-year-old senior dog. I love my grey muzzle, and I am here to tell you old age is not a disease. However, it does require my people to be aware of my special needs, which isn't always easy for them.

You see, because dogs have been domesticated for thousands of years, we have retained an instinct from our wilder days to hide weakness. This instinct does not serve us well in your human environment, where you respond to clear, vocal expressions of discomfort. When you feel ill, you can easily let somebody know about it. We "say" nothing, and you probably won't even notice our age-related changes until we are in extreme pain. Unfortunately, we cannot cry tears or tell you that we are hurting, and even if we could, we try to put up a brave front. Although I am really good at communicating to people when I am happy, hungry, excited or when I want to get their attention, I try to hide my pain in order to make my caretaker, Jenny, feel as if everything is fine. I wag my tail sometimes, not because I want to, but to make her happy.

I became an "official" senior about the time I turned seven years of age, and I became geriatric at 10. Initially, I started feeling pain in my back and legs. My daily activities started to become more difficult, and my body would feel really stiff, especially in the mornings. I just didn't have my usual vigor, and I wasn't interested in playing or going on walks like I used to. I began to sleep a lot more and I stopped enthusiastically waking Jenny in the mornings.

Now, sometimes in the morning, I pant and even drool excessively. I often whimper, and my ears will flatten when someone touches my back-end, because I am sensitive there.

When we dogs are in severe and chronic pain, it affects our lives and overall well being, just as it does for you when you are in pain. We may whine, limp, refuse touch, tuck our tail under us, get a fixed stare, tremble, stop eating or salivate while standing over the food dish, or refuse to get up and move around or drink water.

I sometimes feel hot and feverish when my pain is severe. When this happens, I don't want to eat or drink anything.

We may also shake our heads, rub a body part with our paw, or arch our backs while standing or walking when we are in pain. You may notice that your dog's head or tail is off center as he stands or walks. Some dogs will also hide under furniture or outside away from you when they are in severe pain.

That is the case with me today. I'm in a lot of pain, and I can feel it darting in my hips when I move and even grinding in my joint sockets. I am a pretty mellow guy, but at the moment, I'm anxious and want to be left alone. "C'mon, Claude," a kind voice says, but I cannot move from my dog bed right now; I am just in too much pain. I feel a tug at my collar pulling me up, and the pain is excruciating, so I growl and show my teeth to communicate my displeasure. A good clue that we dogs are in pain is when we have a sudden change in temperament like that. Some of us start showing signs of anxiety and fearfulness. We might change from our normally docile selves to suddenly become aggressive or even start biting. Or the opposite may happen. We might uncharacteristically start withdrawing from you and get very quiet.

In my heart, I am still that carefree, fun-loving puppy I have always been. I have a job, actually lots of them. I am the protector for my family, and it is my job to keep the squirrels out of the yard as well as any other animal that invades it. I used to be able to chase them for hours; however, now my body just won't keep up with my duties. This is hard to get used to, as dogs need jobs, and I will soon have to give up this one to my new friend, Bubba. He is much younger and has my past vigor. That's okay, as my favorite job is "official greeter" anyway. I can still do that just fine.

It is very frustrating for me when I can't physically do what I want to do. I long to chase a ball or Frisbee, and in my heart, I am still that dog. I just don't have the stamina for it anymore, and it feels as if my body is betraying me.

New issues come up nearly every day. Incontinence, for example, often occurs in older dogs. One day, I could not quite make it out of the door in time. I did not make a mess intentionally, and it was very embarrassing for me. Also, my stomach is not what it used to be; I used to be able to eat literally anything, from sticks to bones. I am not eating or digesting my usual food like I used to. Jenny took me to the vet, and he gave me some wonderful pills along with a bit of canned pumpkin to put in my bland food. The pumpkin not only tastes good, but it helps calm my stomach and bowel issues. I did struggle with the pill-taking, but then Jenny put the pills in my favorite treat, hotdogs! That did the trick!

Even though I am eating less lately, I seem to be a lot bigger around the middle. I used to have a waist; now I kinda look like the coffee table. My metabolism has changed as I've gotten older, and I am not running around and going on long walks like I used to.

As with people, obesity in dogs can lead to diabetes, heart problems, arthritis, hip dysplasia and, of course, a shortened life span. My people recently put me on a reduced calorie diet, with chicken broth added to my food for flavor. In addition, I get less treats than I used to now. Instead, they give me frozen green beans and apple pieces for snacks. I actually really like the green beans. I think keeping my weight down will help me get around easier, as the larger I get, the harder it seems to be. I can feel the added weight as I climb the stairs, and squeezing through the dog door is not as quick and easy as it used to be.

I also get more anxious than I used to and sometimes inadvertently do things to upset my people. I feel nervous, for example, when I can see Jenny's mouth moving but don't know what she is saying. The sound is often muffled now. I depend upon body language more, as my hearing is starting to fade over time. The use of hand signals from my people is very helpful now.

My vision is also not what it used to be, and gradually I have had more trouble seeing things, even around the house. When Jenny moves furniture, I have difficulty navigating the room, so I appreciate it when she keeps things the same in the rooms where I spend most of my time.

I really need a soft bed or something comfortable to lie on, as it feels good to my aching body. It's great that Jenny has put cushy bedding around the house in the rooms I like to hang out in. Jenny elevated my main bed just a bit to make it easier for me to get in and out. She also raised my food and water dishes up so I don't have to bend my neck, and that has helped reduce my neck and back pain. Jenny sometimes uses a harness to help lift me up into the car. A towel works, too, and it helps to alleviate pain and makes the process much easier for me.

Slippery floors can be difficult for me, so Jenny trims my nails and the hair around my paws regularly, and she places skid-free rugs in spots where I commonly walk. I love to wear skid-resistant socks on my paws! I also love that she has put fresh water in different rooms around the house so I don't have to walk so far to get a drink.

The older I have gotten, the less I groom myself like I used to. My fur often becomes a bit dull and even matted. Regular brushing and grooming by Jenny is an important part of my life now. I love to be brushed, but my first reaction is to pull away for fear that it will hurt. (When dogs are in pain, we often indicate that we are suffering by giving subtle clues like this as to where the pain is.) The thinning of my coat often causes me to get cold faster. I like to wear a sweater in the winter, especially outside. In the summer, though, I am more prone to heat stress issues. I prefer to rest in a shady area when outside in the summertime, and I don't like to exercise too much then. I appreciate fresh, cool water, especially when it is hot outside.

I used to love being around small children and toddlers. I would chase them around and let them crawl all over me. Now, they tend to scare me and get on my nerves. I get angry sometimes when I am disturbed, and I just don't have the strength to play with them like I used to. My brain is undergoing changes, not unlike human brains do as they age, so my personality is changing as well.

When Jenny accepted me into her life, she made an unspoken contract to protect and care for me. I did the same for her. Yes, my body is changing, but believe me, it's not all bad. Like most senior dogs, I am a wonderful companion and have a lot to offer.

Jenny and I want to help other senior dogs live better lives. That is why we are offering you this book. In the following pages, 20 canine professionals from around the country will pass on the information you will need to help your dog make the most of the years he has left.

No other book on dog care contains the accumulated knowledge and experience of this group of people who dedicate their lives to the care and betterment of senior dogs. We hope you make good use of their advice!

Claude is an official Senior Spokesdog. He has a long life to draw upon and his professional experiences include: Family Protector, Official Greeter, Squirrel Chaser, Foot Warmer, Floor Cleaner and Snuggler. Claude is an expert on the body changes senior dogs go through and the signs and signals they give people.

Below, Jenny and her team have put together a variety of my favorite resources.

Books:

Walks With Sierra – The Story of an Old Soul by Liz Brooking

When Animals Speak by Penelope Smith

The Legacy of Beezer and Boomer–Lessons on Living and Dying from my Canine Brothers by Doug Koktavy

Rescuing Sprite – A Dog Lover's Story by Mark R. Levin

The Nature of Animal Healing by Martin Goldstein

The Holistic Health Guide by Doug Knueven

Canine Body Language: A Photographic Guide to Interpreting the Native Language of the Domestic Dog by Brenda Alof

Senior Dog Books: *www.SeniorDogBooks.com*

Resources and Dog Blogs:

www.DogTime.com

www.AllThingsDogsBlog.com

www.BlogPaws.com

www.PetBytes.org

www.SeniorDogBooks.com/Blog

www.ILoveDogs.com

www.DogForum.com

News & Information:

www.MyDogSpace.com

www.Dogster.com

Pet Products:

www.LovingPetProducts.com

2

Senior Dog Basics with
Jennifer Kachnic, CCMT, CRP

How will I know if my dog is in pain?
How often should my senior dog get veterinary checkups?

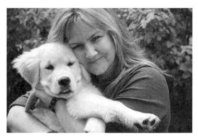

You love your dogs and you trust them to love you–unconditionally. They always forgive you, comfort you and take your side, even when you are wrong. They don't criticize you, and most of all, they think more of you than you think of yourself.

Human companionship is more important to them than even the company of other dogs; they know you can provide the care for them that they need. They are creatures of great kindness and character, and you would benefit from emulating their sense of compassion and forgiveness, their ability to live in the moment and to offer the unconditional love they have always shown to you. When they become senior dogs, we need to return to them all that they have given to us through the years. Remember, they still love and enjoy life even when they don't feel as they used to. Dogs live in the moment and enjoy and relish it all.

Dogs age much faster than people, and their life spans depend greatly upon their size. A year does not seem like a long time, but is equivalent to four to five human years. In general, the larger the breed or size of the dog, the shorter the life span. Smaller dogs generally become senior around the age of 10-12 and the largest breeds around 6-7. Dogs are considered senior in the last 25 percent of their lives. Those are the years they start slowing down, becoming less active and sleeping more. These changes often come with age, but they also can be signs of conditions that might benefit from treatment. Senior dogs can suffer from some of the same disorders as people do.

> *The primary form of communication for dogs is body language.*

It is important that you learn more about this language, especially if you are caring for senior dogs, in order to understand their changing needs. Notice the signs and signals that indicate pain and discomfort. Not only will it save your dog from suffering, it is also much more effective and less costly to detect illness or injury early on in your senior dog. Once you master this language, you will see that your dog communicates with you and others non-stop.

Overt signals that something might be wrong are: vomiting, loss of appetite, weight loss or gain, coughing, sneezing, discharge from the nose, eye or ears, shortness of breath, stool changes, urine color or changes, strong odor in the mouth, hair loss, lumps on the body and changes in skin color. Dogs will also guard a part of their hurting body or rub on furniture when they are in pain. They might limp, undergo changes in their sleep patterns, exhibit difficulty climbing stairs or bark more weakly than they used to. Seriously ill dogs may run a fever or their body temperature could drop to below normal.

If your dog's temperature reaches 105 degrees or above, or drops to 96 degrees or below, take him/her to the vet immediately.

Your dog's respiration rate should normally be around 15-20 breaths per minute (depending on your dog's size) and the pulse should be 80-120 beats per minute when healthy. You can feel a dog's heartbeat by placing you hand on the lower ribcage just behind the elbow. Don't be alarmed if the heartbeat seems irregular compared to a human heartbeat, but you may notice this change if a dog is in pain.

In addition to these relatively obvious physical signs of problems, you will want to look for subtle clues that indicate stress and anxiety in your senior dog. These include the dog putting his tail between his legs, pulling his ears back, stiffening his body, showing teeth, growling and avoiding contact with other humans or dogs.

Other signals of stress include lip-licking, averting their eyes and even yawning. Don't assume your dog is just tired when he yawns, as dogs will also yawn when they feel anxious to help calm themselves down. In addition, dogs might blink their eyes faster than normal, scratch, pant and shake their bodies (as if wet). Excessive drooling could be a response to the presence of food, or it could also be a sign of stress. Grooming in excess—including licking or chewing of paws, legs, tail and genital areas—can also be a sign of anxiety and stress.

Stress can lead to aggressiveness in dogs, which may be another sign that your dog is experiencing difficult physical changes. People find it hard to understand why their dog has suddenly become aggressive to them or others. From the dog's point of view, he is quite vulnerable, with limited means of communication and has no choices in the decisions of his caretaker.

We also need to talk about constipation and diarrhea, both occasionally will occur in older dogs. Incontinence and any unusual bowel issues can also be a sign of a serious health problem in your senior dog, including an infection. Hormone imbalances, loss of bladder muscle control and weak bladder are common in senior dogs. Any bowel movement problem should be discussed with your veterinarian.

Many dogs can start to have dental problems as they age if their teeth are not taken care of properly. When dental issues become serious, all a dog can do is stand over the food bowl and salivate; it is often just too painful to eat. Periodontal disease is one of the most widespread diseases in dogs, and it is estimated that 80% of senior dogs have it. The tissue surrounding a dog's teeth becomes infected and inflamed and can lead to not only bad breath, but major health problems throughout the body.

Seriously ill dogs might also run a fever or their body temperature may drop to below normal.

Foods Are Friends and Foes

Changing their diet may be an option but be sure to make the change gradually. It is not good to constantly switch their foods, but occasionally it can help them stay interested in their diet.

Raw fruits and vegetables can be great healthy low-calorie treats for them but, certain foods should be avoided including raw potatoes as they contain oxalates that can harm the nervous and digestive systems. Grapes, raisins, avocado, ice cream, lemons, tomatoes, onions, garlic, macadamia nuts, nutmeg and persimmons can cause us problems. Chocolate is very toxic to dogs and can even cause death in large quantities. Xylitol in artificial sweeteners can be equally dangerous.

Dogs, of course, love the fat trimmings, but excessive amounts can cause pancreatitis. Chicken bones can be dangerous because of choking. Raw food diets can be a good option along with raw meat bone. However, I do recommend supervision when they eat them.

As Claude mentioned, baby gates are good for keeping dogs out of rooms and attempting to climb stairs you don't want them to climb. There are also pet wheel chairs, ramps and slings you can buy for dogs as well. If you allow them on the couch or bed, pet ramps or doggie stairs will help aid them to easily climb up.

Never leave dogs in a hot car or other hot closed place. The heat rises rapidly and senior dogs, in particular, can suffer from dehydration which can lead to death. If they normally use a kennel, it should be well ventilated during summer months.

Dogs do not deliberately do things to anger you. People often say their dog looks guilty when they have misbehaved. This is not true as that would suggest an advanced level of cognition that is simply not part of their mental process.

To avoid such issues, senior dogs need regular veterinary checkups; twice a year is a good idea at this stage. That may seem like a lot, but remember that because dogs age differently, this is similar to a human senior citizen visiting the doctor every four years. Your veterinarian will screen for health problems typical of older dogs, and you can get your dog the help he needs early on. The last few decades have shown an increased life span for pets because veterinary science, as well as alternative therapies, has made such great strides.

Any change in appetite or bowel movements can be a sign of a potential problem.

Talk with your veterinarian about age-related health problems, alternative therapies and the preventative steps you can take to ensure a long and healthy life for your old friend.

Jennifer Kachnic has spent her life working and volunteering in animal welfare including fostering hundreds of dogs for local shelters through the years. She is a Certified Therapy Dog Handler for the American Humane Society, Certified Animal Reiki Practitioner and a Certified Canine Massage Therapist. She has been a regular contributor to a variety of pet magazines including Animal Wellness, Mile High Dog Magazine *and* Bark.

As President of The Grey Muzzle Organization, she leads volunteers around the country working to provide grants to animal shelters and rescues nationwide for senior dog programs.

SeniorDogBooks.com
PO Box 3331, Littleton, CO 80161
303-324-3911
Jenny@SeniorDogBooks.com

Facebook: Jennifer.Kachnic
Twitter: SeniorDogBooks
Blog: GreyMuzzle.org/Blog

In addition to Claude's favorite resources, here are mine as well:

My Favorite Resources

ASPCA – Animal Control Center
www.ASPCA.com
Humane Society of Veterinary Medical Association
www.HSVMA.org
American Humane Association
www.AmericanHumane.org
Holistic Veterinarian List
www.HolisticVetList.com
Senior Dog Books
www.SeniorDogBooks.com
Dog News and Information
www.DogTipper.com
www.PetPlace.com
Holistic Supplements for Dogs
www.HolisticPetInfo.com

Dog Blogs
www.BlogPaws.com
www.BlogPark.com
www.SeniorDogBooks.com/Blog
www.AllThingsDogsBlog.com

The Holistic Guide by Doug Knueven DVM, CVA,
Caring for your Aging Dog by Alof, Brenda
The Living Well Guide for Senior Dogs by Diane Morgan
    and Wayne Hunthausen, DVM
The Nature of Animal Healing by Martin Goldstein, DVM
When Your Best Friend Becomes Your Old Friend
    by Gina Stewart, Don and Kellie Rainwater

3

The Benefits of Having A Senior Dog in Your Life

Are there actually health benefits for people who have a senior dog in their life?

Where can I go to adopt a senior dog?

Imagine for a moment that you are a dog. You're fortunate to have met your lifelong companion and soul mate. Whether watching TV, going to the beach, snuggling in bed together, or just getting out for a quick ride in the car to run some errands, you find the joy in just being together and sharing your life with that trusted friend. Imagine now, that you've awakened one morning to find that this person on whom you depend for your every comfort and necessity is now gone. As will happen to each of us, he or she has passed away.

All of a sudden, there is chaos in your home. Strange people are everywhere and the stress is palpable. Somebody leashes you up and takes you for a ride. You arrive in an unfamiliar place to be greeted by a cacophony of noise. Barking and distress cries reverberate off hard surfaces. You're led down a long hallway and into a room where you are left alone. There are no blankets, no

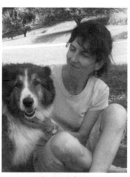

Liz Booking

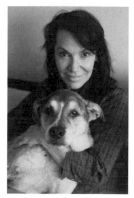

Sherri Franklin

toys and the floor is cold cement still damp from urine and disinfectant. You're afraid and confused and you've just lost your loved one—the person who was there for you. Is this really what he intended for you?

Sadly, this traumatizing ordeal is a fairly typical scenario experienced by tens of thousands of senior dogs whose guardians simply had no plan for them upon their death. In other circumstances, significant changes to a guardian's living arrangement, or economic, employment or health status are the catalysts for the ultimate displacement of a beloved family dog.

All too often, when the elderly are faced with the difficult decision to move to an assisted living facility, they are also told that their dog is not welcome. At a time when, quite frankly, they need its company more than ever, their four-legged companion is barred from the facility. Finally, many older dogs used as breeding machines by unscrupulous puppy mills will find themselves homeless when the operation is shut down or the dog is deemed no longer useful.

San Francisco-based Muttville Senior Dog Rescue has saved more than 1,000 senior dogs from situations just like these. Some of their more fortunate rescues had known great love. Others never had the opportunity. Each, however, had the capacity to give and receive it in abundance and, whether fostered until death or adopted, they were among the lucky few to be given a second chance at life and the opportunity to thrive in a safe and loving home environment.

The need for senior dog adoption is great. What makes each of the circumstances creating this need even more saddening is the fact that, despite the wonderful attributes of older dogs and all the best efforts of most shelters, these dogs are frequently overlooked in favor of puppies and younger animals. The ageism that causes seniors to be passed over is a prejudice without merit, as oftentimes it's the older dog that is best suited for a happy household and a lasting marriage of dog and family.

What You See Is What You Get

With an older dog, what you see is what you get. There are no surprises. Their physical size is established so there are no mysteries about whether they'll exceed the weight limit for your apartment, and by and large, their temperament and personality are also fully developed. In other words, they've become what and who they are going to be.

Of course, you can expect that your dog's confidence will blossom as he adjusts to his new surroundings and the trauma of his loss is replaced by the reassurance of knowing that you are there for him. Beyond that, however, his demeanor will be evident in a first meeting, allowing you to fairly size up how he will fit into both your lifestyle and the family dynamic.

Most Older Dogs Have Already Been Trained

An older dog has typically had some basic obedience training and is already familiar with the essential commands that will make life enjoyable for both of you (Come. Sit. Stay.). Equally important, he is more than likely also housetrained, unlike his puppy counterpart. If your household includes very young children, you will welcome the fact that you will not have to endure housetraining and potty training all at the same time.

That said; don't believe the adage, "An old dog can't learn new tricks." It's simply not true. If there is a special need and you are so inclined, these old dogs are eager to please and enjoy the attention and mental stimulation that your training sessions can provide.

The Older Dog is Past His Chewing Phase

To anyone who has ever had his favorite shoes, the furniture, an heirloom rug, or the baseboards of his house chewed with endless abandon, rejoice! This is typical puppy behavior but not at all what to expect from a normal, adult dog.

A Senior Dog Requires Less Exercise

Let's face it, as we age we all slow down a bit. You can expect an older dog to be less frisky and rambunctious than his younger counterparts, and in most cases, his requirement for exercise will be far less. This attribute alone makes the older dog a great fit for many family situations and an ideal match for the aging adult as well.

The Perfect Match: Pairing Seniors with Seniors

As they age, like each of us, dogs will have health issues that need to be addressed. Many of these common ailments are addressed in the other chapters of this book so we'll focus here on the benefits of adopting a senior dog instead—and they are many, especially for aging adults.

Exercise

What better excuse to fire up the muscles and get outside than to walk the dog. A dog's need to regularly relieve himself and sniff his way around the neighborhood is a great way to get the elderly out of doors, moving joints and muscles, and enabling them to see the beauty around them. Never again will they miss a beautiful sunset, the fall leaves as they change color, or the first signs of spring. Having a dog makes one live in the present and focus on the now.

Companionship

For some reason, a dog creates an invitation to talk. Walking a dog is a great way to meet one's neighbors and to build community. For some reason, the wag of a tail has done more to break down social barriers and build friendships than anything we know.

As an aside, dogs are also great listeners. They are known to keep secrets and act positively enchanted even if your singing is slightly off key.

Those of us who have been lucky enough to hold a warm dog in our arms, or share the couch or a bed with one, know the benefits of simply listening to the sound his breath. The sound of a dog breathing has a calming effect.

> *Studies show the health benefits of having a pet. Among those benefits is a distinct lowering of blood pressure and anxiety. We're not surprised. Are you sold yet?*

Success Stories

One could continue to wax on and on about the benefits of adopting an older dog, but those who have experienced it first-hand are far more convincing, so we've included a few stories to reinforce why it may just be the best thing you'll ever do.

Donna's Calling

At 68-years of age, Donna is still in her prime. In her garage you'll find the shell of an RV-4, a two-seater airplane she is building and intends to fly next spring, and an old car, which upon closer inspection appears to be used far more frequently for napping by her Lhasa Apso, Callie, than for any transportation.

Callie is just one of the handfuls of geriatric dogs that share Donna's lovely ½-acre plot of land in California replete with roses and dotted with Gravenstein apple trees, an organic vegetable garden, and a magnificent clutch of laying hens. Once found wandering the streets of rural California, Callie was covered in burrs and her fur was so matted around her eyes that she could not see. Now 11-year old Callie is living the good life.

We enter Donna's ranch-style home to find the rest of her charges: Ollie, a 13-year old Cocker Spaniel, who is clearly head of this household, and Olive, an older Labrador, who simply holds court from a fleece bed strategically placed so that she can follow all the activities of the house.

Recent foster Dorrey, a sweet, black Pekingese enters the room looking totally content and fully adjusted to the paradise in which she now finds herself after weeks in a hot, Merced-based shelter.

No stranger to dogs, Donna trained and showed her Welsh Pembroke Corgi to his championship some decades ago. Today, she chooses instead to share her life with this group of seniors, including a 14-year old Corgi rescue named Maddie who follows her around the house with a spring in his step that belies his advanced age.

As she leads us through her beautiful garden, dogs in tow, she shares with a chuckle her mother's words, "Don't plant anything that doesn't give you anything back." I am struck by how those words are such an apt metaphor for Donna's life, and one that completely explains why she continues to take in and care for senior dogs. They are so grateful— and one can easily see the happiness and purpose that tending to these dogs has given her. As she says, "It was a calling," and one she is lucky to have answered.

The Object of His Affection: Ivan's Story

Ivan, an 83-year old widowed and retired school teacher, is another participant in Muttville's very successful initiative to pair senior dogs with senior citizens. The miniature Schnauzer with which Ivan had shared a full life passed away years ago. Losing this special and steadfast companion left a gaping hole in Ivan's life so he decided to do something about it.

Just about that time, an 11-year old mini Schnauzer was surrendered to a shelter in Bakersfield, California. Neglect and abandonment had left this once beautiful dog now covered with ticks and fleas. As it has so many times before, Muttville stepped in to take the dog, knowing that given her age she would be on the short list for euthanasia. That was the first bit of luck for this lovely gal named MacEnzie. A second stroke of luck was soon to arrive when Ivan contacted Muttville.

Housetrained? Yes. She loves to cuddle? Yes. MacEnzie was all of those things and more. This was the dog for him! Ivan was able to find the perfect match, a new best friend, and a focus for all of his energies. MacKenzie has happily settled into her forever home and Ivan is absolutely delighted. He reports that she commands all of his attention and that he gives it willingly. That makes both of them very, very happy.

For seniors on a fixed income, the prospect of dog ownership is something to consider. For that reason, Muttville Senior Dog Rescue facilitates its senior adoptions by underwriting the adoption fees and funding a *New Dog Care Kit* courtesy of the Pedigree Foundation whose Innovation Grant helps support this effort.

Old and Young: Happy Together

Senior dogs aren't just for seniors. Becky, her three-year old daughter and husband already knew this from past experience. After losing their previous dog to old age several months prior, this young family felt incomplete. Seeing Phoebe on Muttville's web site was all it took to convince them that a meeting was in order.

Phoebe, a Corgi and Border Collie mix has a backstory that is all too familiar. Temporarily housed at Animal Care and Control (ACC) of Orange County, California she was in bad shape. At the age of 12, deaf in both ears, and with most of her teeth literally rotting away, she was passed over for adoption. ACC called Muttville to save her from certain death and shortly thereafter Phoebe arrived in San Francisco, care of one of the many volunteer transporters across the country who provide this vital service in the placement of dogs.

A short stint with one of the "fosters" in the Muttville network put Phoebe on track to leading a happier life. This dear old girl was given the healthcare and dental work she desperately needed to bring back the sparkle in her eyes and that's when her circumstance changed for the better.

Now at home with a big backyard, a little sister to protect and play with, and a mom intent on teaching her sign language to overcome the issues associated with her hearing loss, this old mutt is one happy dog.

Phoebe is absolutely adored by her new family and the feeling is mutual. Not a day goes by without a belly rub or two, a walk to the park, and a meal lovingly prepared by a mother who cares for both of her girls, two and four-legged, with tender purpose.

Sherri Franklin has been involved in animal welfare for more than 20 years and is the founder and Executive Director of Muttville Senior Dog Rescue. As vice chair of the Animal Control and Welfare Commission of San Francisco for six years, she co-authored the backyard dog ordinance setting minimum standards for dogs kept outside, and helped to get the city's remaining aging elephants out of the zoo and into a sanctuary. Sherri has received a commendation from the City of San Francisco, the Guardian Award from In Defense of Animals (IDA), and the prestigious Jefferson Award in recognition of her community and public service on behalf of animals.

Liz Brooking is the author of the blog and award-winning book Walks With Sierra.

Muttville Senior Dog Rescue
PO Box 410207
San Francisco, CA 94141
www.Muttville.org

Where to Find Your Senior Dog

There are many animal shelters across the country but few fill the desperate need to place senior dogs. The following list is an excellent starting point for your research. Keep in mind that each of these organizations needs volunteers to survive and funding to underwrite their noble efforts.

If you're not yet ready to adopt your senior, consider becoming a foster parent, a dog walker, or providing some other service or donation that will help ease the suffering of an old dog and provide him with a shot at a new beginning and the happy ending he deserves.

West Coast

Muttville Senior Dog Rescue, San Francisco, CA
www.Muttville.org
or *https://www.facebook.com/Muttville.Senior.Dog.Rescue*

Old Dog Haven, Lake Stevens, WA
www.OldDogHaven.org

Seniors for Seniors Program, Seattle, WA
www.SrDogs.com
www.AnimalShelter.org

H.A.R.T. (Humane Animal Rescue Team) Fillmore, CA
www.HumaneAnimalRescueTeam.com

Senior Mutt Match, San Diego, CA
www.WeCareToo.com

Central

The Sanctuary for Senior Dogs, Cleveland, OH
www.SanctuaryForSeniorDogs.org

Central Texas Dachshund Rescue, Austin, TX
http://www.ctdr.org/hospice.html

St. Louis Senior Dogs Project, St. Louis, MO
www.SrDogs.com
www.STLSeniorDogProject.org

Pets for Seniors, Peoria, IL
www.PetsForSeniors.org

Denver Dumb Friends League, Denver, CO
www.DDFL.com

East Coast

Out to Pasture, Newington, CT
www.OutToPasture.org

North Shore Animal League, Port Washington, NY
www.AnimalLeague.org

National

Petfinder
http://www.PetFinder.com/index.html

Pet Harbor – National list of pets available for adoption
www.PetHarbor.com
www.HowToChooseYourDog.com

Pet Guardian Angel of America–
Information to assist in pet matches for your lifestyle
www.PSAA.com

Adopting a Pet Information

www.AdoptAPet.com

4

Common Canine Geriatric Diseases with Brian Lapham DVM, CVA

What symptoms should I look for in my dog?

What can I do to make the veterinarian appointments more productive?

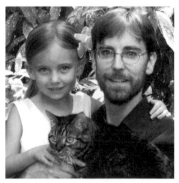

Looking into the eyes of my 16-year-old Golden Retriever, I knew that his soul was still running and playing. His young bark, so vibrant and piercing, his head held with a slight tilt that invited a romp. His body, however, was showing the signs of the inevitable aging process. His coordination slightly off, joints stiff, vision and hearing starting to go. He had given me so much over the years–undying devotion, immediate reaction to the words "go for a walk?" and a very furry belly to rub that could overcome the worst of my days. Now it was my turn. My place to make this world a little easier for him, more comfortable, and if needed, a peaceful ending.

As a veterinarian for the last 12 years, and a pet lover for my entire life (I have pictures to prove it!), I have learned a lot about pet health care. With absolutely no exception, my biggest lessons have come through my aging patients. I have been taught how to gently assist an arthritic pet without embarrassing them, how to soften food for sore gums without it dribbling down their chest and simple techniques, such as keeping the stair lights on to assist their way at night.

Below are some of the more common issues with our geriatric pets, symptoms to look for, treatment options, and most importantly, ways to prevent, or at least slow down, the progression of these issues.

Dental Disease

Misty was a 12-year-old Labrador mix that came to me for her annual wellness exam. She was eating well, but didn't seem as interested in her hard treats. Her physical exam was unremarkable, until it came time to look in her mouth. Moderate to severe gingivitis was present along her entire gumline with at least one tooth likely infected. I say likely, because I could not see most of her teeth due to the amount of tartar and calculus present! My client and I discussed Misty's dental issues, and my client reluctantly chose to perform a thorough dental cleaning and evaluation. She, of course, was concerned about the risks of anesthesia and Misty's advanced age. I assured her that Misty would be well taken care of and monitored throughout the procedure.

On the day of Misty's dental cleaning, she had blood drawn in advance of the procedure, an intravenous catheter with fluids started, modern anesthetics administered and a thorough dental cleaning with intraoral radiographs. While undergoing the procedure, Misty's vital signs were constantly monitored, including blood pressure, ECG, heart and respiratory rates, oxygen and carbon dioxide levels. During the dental cleaning and evaluation, we found two severely infected teeth that we surgically extracted. Misty returned home that evening and by morning was nearly back to her old self. One week later, I got a call from my client to report that Misty was not only back to her old self, but better than before! It is amazing what taking pain and infection away will do to your demeanor!

How often do we really look in their mouths? Brush daily? Provide proper chew bones—which they actually use? Not as often as we probably should. Not surprisingly then, if there is one problem that almost every one of my aged patients (and many younger) have, it is dental disease. This is a shame, because in comparison to some of the other afflictions that befall our aging friends, dental disease is the easiest diagnosis in the world. All you have to do is open up your pet's mouth and take a look. A really good look—pulling the lips back into a smile, so you can see all the way into those back molars. The easy way to decide if there is a problem is to imagine that this is your mouth.

- Are there signs of gingivitis?
- Tartar or calculus (calcified tartar)?
- How about loose or missing teeth?
- Are roots exposed(ouch!!)?
- What do you smell?
- Is there a strong odor that is more than just dog breath?

If any of these symptoms are present, ask yourself this: would you want your mouth to look like this? I suspect not. Dental disease isn't just a cosmetic problem; in advanced cases, your pet may not want to eat hard food or treats, may act restless at night or even have a soft bulge over the base of their cheek bone, a result of a tooth abscess.

Treatment for dental disease starts with a systematic evaluation of all of the animal's teeth. This is done with intraoral radiographs, scaling and polishing of all teeth and treatment of any existing dental disease all of which are done while your pet is under general anesthesia. Proper evaluation of dental disease below the gum line simply is not possible without anesthesia—sedation is not enough.

Anesthesia, especially of older animals, is an understandable concern for all pet guardians. As veterinarians, we, too, are always mindful of the risks associated with all anesthetic procedures. Thankfully though, with the advent of modern anesthetics and monitoring equipment, the risk of anesthetic adverse events are very rare, with one study indicating a mere 0.05 percent risk to dogs. Compare that to the risk of infection, tooth loss and pain associated with untreated dental disease, which is essentially 100 percent in our aged animals ... I think the lesser of the evils is pretty obvious.

Despite the fact that treating dental disease is usually successful in clearing up any problems, prevention of dental disease in the first place is certainly the preferable route I encourage my clients to take. Simple measures such as treating dental conditions early on can prevent dental pain and tooth loss further down the road.

> *Daily brushing of all teeth, using a finger brush or soft-headed child's toothbrush, is recommended. Good chew toys–such as raw carrots, edible bones meant for dental health and chew ropes can be very helpful in removing dental plaque and strengthen gum tissue.*

It goes without saying that these chew toys must only be used under supervision at all times, and the pets chewing habits must be taken into account. A very strong and determined chewer should not be given the same chew toys as the older Chihuahua!

Osteoarthritis

One of my favorite patients, Hannah, came to me originally for euthanasia. She was an older boxer, with many small issues in her life that, all together, were causing her quality of life to suffer. Upon examination and review of her extensive history, I noticed that nothing had been done to address her known arthritic joints. I was told by her folks that she was too old to handle medication and with her other issues it was not worth treating that condition. I pleaded with them to at least give me a chance to see if I could improve her quality of life through a multi-modal approach centered around pain relief.

With their agreement, we started Hannah on a regimen of supplements, massage, home-based physical therapy and pain medication.

A week later, I received a phone call from my clients telling me that Hannah was doing much better and that her appetite and demeanor had returned to normal. It took us another month of adjusting medication and continuing home therapies before we all felt Hannah was back to her old self. Hannah went on to live another 4 years—happy, comfortable, active and a perpetual book-chewer, her only vice.

If we all live long enough, we will all probably suffer from one form or another of arthritis. In fact, 90 percent of Americans will have some level of arthritis by the age of 40! Unfortunately, so will many of our pets. Arthritis is an inflammation of a joint, due to many different causes including trauma, infection, degeneration or metabolic reasons. Most often we deal with age-related degeneration or osteoarthritis. This is a wearing and thinning of the cartilage in the joint, leading to bone spurs and cysts that induce inflammation and pain.

The diagnosis of osteoarthritis is often made by patient history and physical exam. Radiographs (x-ray) can help determine severity and location, but they do not often tell us the whole story, since cartilage— the main victim of osteoarthritis—cannot be seen on x-ray (more advanced imaging such as CT or MRI exams could be utilized, but it is rare in veterinary medicine). For this reason, it is important that owners be aware of even small changes in their pet's mobility and appearance.

Early on in the process of developing arthritis, the signs can be quite subtle. A stiffness first thing in the morning or after a long rest, having to "warm up" into an activity, or not being as interested in a long walk or prolonged play-period. As the disease progresses, limping in a joint after activity, refusing to do any type of exercise, or loss of muscle mass may be noted.

In the end stage, our pets can be in pain even without activity, have a significant decreased mobility in the joint and need assistance with simple activities such as squatting to go to the bathroom. Externally, you may notice a soft swelling over the joint. If you bend the joint, it may feel stiff to you, or even uncomfortable to your pet. A veterinarian will notice more subtle signs such as decreased range of motion, crepitus (snapping and popping of the joint as it is manipulated), soft tissue swelling and discomfort.

Treatments for osteoarthritis range from simple supplements to radical surgery, depending on the severity of the condition. Treatments include:

- Neutraceutical supplements should be included in the treatment regime for all osteoarthritic patients that can tolerate them. Glucosamine, fish oil and MSM all have benefits to the joints. In addition, herbals such as Boswellia and turmeric, have been used for many generations to treat the symptoms of osteoarthritis.

- Physical therapy to help increase range of motion and build muscle mass has also been shown to be very helpful when treating pets that are suffering from osteoarthritis.

- Alternative therapies such as acupuncture and spinal manipulation have benefits.

- Drug therapy to control pain is necessary in some patients to keep them active and improve their quality of life.

- In end-stage arthritic patients, surgery can be beneficial—modern medicine has made total hip replacements almost routine, and we are perfecting knee and elbow replacements as you read this.

The most important treatment (in addition to being a preventative measure) is to have the pet lose any excess weight. Any extra pounds the patient carries puts additional stress on the joints and can make symptoms worse.

Preventing osteoarthritis is more challenging. Certainly controlling excessive amounts of weight, through the use of appropriate amounts of food and exercise, before there is an issue is the most ideal approach. Currently there is healthy debate among veterinarian doctors as to whether supplementation or herbals early on in a pet's life can have a protective benefit further down the road. I often recommend either fish oil or glucosamine to my arthritis-prone breed patients early in their life, as these supplements have little to no side effect and are inexpensive. Worse-case scenario, they don't prevent arthritis at all, but at least they will be present in the body the day they are needed rather than six months later when we identify the joint problem.

Sensory Loss

Murphy was an older miniature poodle that came to see me for his annual wellness exam. His elderly caretakers did not know how old he was, but to say he was as old as the hills was an understatement! He had lived with my clients for the last 10 years. As Murphy ambled into the exam room, he continued right by me and walked full-on into the opposite door. As I watched Murphy go by, I could see his completely opaque cataracts–this little guy could not see a hand in front of his face. I then asked his folks how long he had been blind.

To my surprise they were taken aback by the question and stated that he could see just fine! Murphy of course was completely blind, but had fooled his owners into believing he could see by learning the layout of his home, and knowing how to maneuver without hindrance. Everything was fine until Murphy came into a new situation—like my examination room. Murphy was not the least bit put out by his lack of vision and is a perfect example of how amazingly adaptable my patients can be.

For the sake of simplicity and space, I have lumped many of the sensory problems that our aging pets suffer from into one category–simply called sensory loss. Sensory perception is the way our pets interpret the world around them–using smell, hearing, vision, taste and touch. Our pets are very much "in the moment" creatures. They require these sensory inputs to understand what is happening around them. Subsequently, as the senses start to fail, our pet's interpretation of the world around them is altered and may even affect their quality of life. Often, there is not a lot we can do about the declining sensory perception our older pets suffer from, we can help them by improving what is left of their senses, and to help compensate for the loss when their senses are gone altogether. Lucky for me, my patients are much more adaptable to these kinds of conditions than we two-legged creatures!

The symptoms of sensory loss can be quite varied depending on which sense is affected and the severity of loss. Vision loss often starts with a pet having difficulty seeing in dim light–perhaps tripping on the stairs at night or getting lost in a dark room or back yard. Hearing changes can include "ignoring" you while being called or looking in the wrong direction. Taste and smell are integrally related, often reported by the owner as a "pickiness" with foods–preferring soft foods, warmed or table foods over their regular kibble. Touch is really a combination of several issues–balance, conscious proprioception and nervous input. Losses in touch sensation are often seen as the pet being unsteady while walking, especially when turning or attempting quick movements, and uncertainty on irregular surfaces.

There are some simple ways to help our pets compensate for sensory loss.

- Good lighting, particularly in areas where there are steps or obstacles, is an easy way to help a senior pet who is having difficulties with sight.

- With hearing issues, clicker training or using a deep voice can be helpful as often times pets can still hear those frequencies even as their hearing of other frequencies diminishes. In addition, since your pet may not respond to commands, it is not advisable to allow them off-leash in unsecured areas.

- Loss of taste and smell senses can be easily compensated for by using foods with strong flavors and smells, warming them up to release some of those odors, and adding a small amount of water or broth to the food. Putting small amounts of unique table foods such as chicken, sardines, cheese or hamburger in their food can also increase the palatability without unbalancing the diet.

Summary

There are many other conditions that occur in our aging pets–from senility and incontinence issues, to devastating diseases like cancer. Having yearly and even 6-month thorough examinations with your veterinarian, especially one that enjoys working with senior pets, can be extremely important to catch these conditions early, or better yet, to prevent them. A few tips to make that appointment more productive are:

1. Make sure to have plenty of time during the visit–arrive a few minutes early to fill out any paperwork, and ask for at least a 30-minute appointment–longer if there are multiple issues.

2. Write down any questions or concerns you might have, as it makes for a more efficient visit but also prevents you from forgetting to ask anything.

3. Bring all of your medication bottles and current dosing information.

4. If you are new to this particular practice or have not met the veterinarian before, consider making an appointment for a "meet and greet". This allows you to interview the veterinarian to see if you both have similar philosophies.

Now, go out there and enjoy your seniors! You know they are waiting for you—on the couch of course....

Brian Lapham is a Doctor of Veterinarian Medicine based in Durham, North Carolina who has a special interest in holistic treatments, such as acupuncture, pain management, Chinese herbs, nutritional counseling, and hospice care. In addition to these holistic treatment options, he also provides traditional care such as dentistry and surgery. He received his veterinary degree from the University of Florida in 1999, and completed a 1 year internship at Gulfcoast Veterinary Referral. Dr. Lapham's acupuncture training was completed at the Chi Institute. Currently, he is the owner of Southpoint Animal Hospital.

Southpoint Animal Hospital
5601 Fayetteville Road
Durham, NC 27713
919-226-0043
drlapham@SouthpointPets.com
www.SouthpointPets.com

My Favorite Resources:

American Animal Hospital Association: *www.Aahanet.org*

Chi Institute: *www.tcvm.com*

Dental information: *www.ToothVet.com*

Arthritis medical info: *www.VeterinaryPartner.com*

Cancer information: *www.cvm.ncsu.edu*

Only Natural Pet Store: *www.OnlyNaturalPet.com*

The Whole Dog Journal: *www.Whole-Dog-Journal.com*

Animal Wellness Magazine: *www.AnimalWellnessMagazine.com*

5

How Senior Dogs Think and Communicate with Terri O'Hara

How do dogs communicate with you?

What do they want you to know?

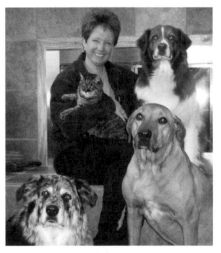

Quality of life is no doubt your number one goal for your senior canine companion. But as your dog ages, physical and emotional changes can leave you questioning how she is truly feeling. You may wonder if the walks are too long, or if the level of play is sufficient. Questions such as these can be explored with the services of an animal communicator.

Through an intuitive consultation, an animal communicator will offer you information from your dog's perspective. These insights provide a deeper understanding of your senior's needs and can ease your job as caregiver, while giving you much-deserved peace of mind.

Professional animal communicators are available throughout the world, serving as advocates of all species of animals. Their services complement your loving care, along with the professional health care of veterinarians and other providers. With this helpful team, your dog is promised an excellent quality of life.

When you work with reputable animal communicators, the information they offer comes from the spirit of your dog. The conversation occurs through intuition, also known as telepathy. The job of the communicator is to listen from the heart and to be open to receiving information from the animal's perspective. That information comes in the form of mental pictures, emotions, physical sensations, energy, and words (although, unlike humans, animals do not use a lot of words). Communicators take everything they sense and put it together like a puzzle to offer a voice for your dog.

You will know quickly whether or not the animal communicator is connecting with your dog. How? It's simple: you will hear information that the communicator could not have known prior to the session.

For example, when a new client called me to talk to Sasha, her 12-year-old German shepherd, she started by asking, "Can you tell me how she is doing generally?" Immediately, I felt happiness, pride, and fatigue. I asked Sasha to explain why she was feeling these emotions. Sasha communicated by sending a visual image, which came into my awareness. She showed me an image of her going out through a door with her human companion, Elizabeth, in the early morning. They turned left at the end of a driveway and stopped at a mailbox, where Sasha sniffed the bush next to the post. Then they walked on toward a street corner, where they turned right and went a couple of blocks to a park. I saw her wagging her tail and holding her head high. She was proud that she could still go for walks.

When I reported this, Elizabeth laughed and said, "This is exactly our routine every morning at 6:30 a.m." Next, Sasha sent me an image of walking much slower on the way back, going into their house, lumbering up to a bright blue, oval-shaped dog bed in front of a sliding glass door and plopping down a bit awkwardly. I then felt fatigue in my own body as a way of sensing her experience. I sent an acknowledgement to Sasha with a feeling of understanding her exhaustion. Based on the level of deep fatigue I felt while communicating, I explained to Elizabeth that I sensed Sasha was tired most of the time, however, the happiness visuals of her walks offered assurance she was saying they were well worth the effort and provided her much joy. Elizabeth believed my information matched the behaviors she witnessed in Sasha. This allowed her to feel comfortable with my services from that point on, trusting the information was truly coming from Sasha.

When working with senior animals, I ask the dog to show me what it feels like to be in his or her body. I use intuitive awareness to gradually scan from head to tail and slowly down each leg. Pain will arise in my own body, in sensations of burning, throbbing, aching, dullness, sharpness, etc., as I focus on each area. For example, I may suddenly feel a dull, strong ache in my left knee. Then, by focusing on the physical sensation, I send a message back to the dog to clarify what I am receiving. Once I feel that the content is confirmed, I share the details with the person. The information gained can then be taken to the health care professionals working with the dog to assist with the medical care. In this way, and others, animal communication can help you lovingly nurture your dog to the final days.

Before you hire the services of an animal communicator, be sure you feel comfortable with the person's background, experience, and reputation. It is important that the person has been working as a professional with clients for a period of time. You decided what length of time feels right to you. Perhaps you may want someone who has at least a year of experience, or more. Also, ask them where they have worked. It's good to find someone that has been offered their services at public events or pet stores. This indicates they are successful with their skills if they are returning to a public venue repeatedly.

Requesting testimonials from a potential communicator can be another way to research and find the best match for you. Ask communicators if they have client references list for you to explore. Another option is to search the internet. You will find a respectable referral list at *www.AnimalTalk.net.*

Finally, in my opinion, personal recommendations from someone you know and trust is an excellent way to find a trustworthy professional animal communicator.

I encourage you to utilize this animal communication service however it best suits you. For instance, you may find it fun to have just one session to gain an overall understanding of the many curiosities you've had about your dog throughout your years together. Or, you may prefer to work more regularly with a communicator in order to gain clarity on various issues that arise as your dog's behavior shifts with age. It is also absolutely fine if you don't believe in the concept of a person tuning in to your dog for a conversation. If it doesn't work for you, don't do it. Being skeptical is completely normal, especially when you try something new that you don't understand. However, if you are curious and find yourself thinking, *I will do anything for my dog*, then you might want to give it a try.

Now, on to what senior dogs have to say…

After working for sixteen years with thousands of families, I've found the most common request for help is to assess senior animals and their quality of life. I have assisted over 500 senior dogs by being their voice to the best of my abilities. I'm always impressed when they share how they are doing in their old dog body. Routinely, when I ask how they feel, I hear a common and powerful message … ***life is good!*** That truly is their motto.

> *Animals are very skillful at living in the present moment.*
> *They don't worry about the past or fret about the future.*
> *Although their past can affect their behaviors, they are not*
> *thinking about it over and over the way humans do.*
> *They are living in the now and encourage you to join them.*

Often, senior dogs find it disturbing when their human companion is worried or anxious about his or her state of being. They wonder why people focus on what might happen in the future rather that what is currently occurring. Your dog's desire is to encourage you to concentrate on the fun you could be having together, rather than on being upset unnecessarily. He thinks in the positive and does his best to get you there, too. Perhaps he brings you toys, nudges your arm, or looks soulfully into your eyes. His message to you is *stick to the moment.*

Another insight I have gained from my communication with senior dogs is that their perception of pain may not be what you imagine. I remember working with a dog named Bud, a big, handsome, Chesapeake Bay retriever mix who had just undergone major knee surgery the week prior. I asked him, "How is your knee?" He replied, "Which one?" I smiled. That was the day I learned to never assume a dog is living in his pain.

Animals are very capable of removing their awareness from the area that hurts. They look away from the pain, so to speak, and instead focus on what feels good. This isn't the same as denial. They simply take their consciousness elsewhere. If a human hurts her elbow, she tells people about it all week long. If a dog hurts her elbow, she immediately figures out ways to play and have fun on her other three legs. Dogs are not just being stoic with their pain, they are being practical. This doesn't mean that they never feel pain. They simply don't dwell on it.

Moving on to an important topic...

Within the loving relationship between you and your dog lies the reality that he or she will leave some day. No one likes to think about it ahead of time, but when the senior years approach, death becomes a glaring certainty. Dying is very difficult to contemplate for humans. This is usually not so for dogs. They do not fear their impending transition. Instead, they embrace it.

Animals teach that death is a process. Aching joints, weakening muscles, and digestive issues are common occurrences for elder dogs. Illnesses can also be components of preparing for end of life. Although they can be challenging for both of you, physical changes are a necessary part of the experience. This process allows your dog to slow down and accept the deterioration of his body so he can begin to welcome the completion of his life. A senior dog does not view a disease as a problem. She embraces anything and everything as a part of her journey. Through my experience, dogs have shown me that they gracefully accept all that is going on within their bodies.

I regularly tell clients with elder animals, "*Death isn't always easy and it isn't always pretty, but it can be peaceful and wonderful.*" Years ago, when I said this during a public presentation, a woman called out from the audience: "Neither is giving birth, but that's beautiful too!" This says it all in a nutshell.

> *We must remember that the journey of life for every being has a beginning, a middle and an end. A birth, a life, a death. Your dog knows this. She is not upset that her life will end, but rather is living life to its fullest until her body simply can no longer go on. When it is too difficult to be in the ailing body, your dog will embrace her state of being and allow her death process to occur.*

Dogs are not afraid to die. So, if you are worried about your dog's death, or you are afraid about life without your dog, be sure to acknowledge that these are your feelings. Be careful to not project them onto your canine friend. Always be honest with your beloved dog, because he already knows what you are thinking and feeling. He can read your thoughts, emotions, and intentions. Don't try to pretend, it will only cause upset and confusion.

I am reminded of the story of a sweet black and tan dachshund named Daisy. Sam and Maureen adopted her when she was a puppy. She enjoyed a life full of love. As she aged, she slowed down bit by bit. After turning 13, she shifted more dramatically. At this point, Maureen became sad all the time. She couldn't stop thinking about the day that she would no longer have Daisy. When cuddling, if she got teary, she would go into another room to cry. When talking with friends about her fear that Daisy would be dying soon, she would change the subject if Daisy walked into the room. Maureen's efforts were to protect the dog she loved so deeply. It didn't work. Daisy began to act depressed.

Sam and Maureen asked me, "Does she need anything, anything at all?" I heard from Daisy the word confused. I deciphered that she couldn't understand why she sensed sadness and regret in the household. The heaviness was burdening her and dampening her joy.

I explained to Daisy that her human companions were concerned for the loss they would experience when she dies. She showed me her elder body wiggling with happiness, picking up balls, waddling along on walks. I explained to them, "She wants you to know she is still alive and having fun." With further discussion, I encouraged them to join her. They promised to change.

Two weeks later, Maureen and Sam called to say the sadness in the household had lifted. They reported that Daisy was perkier than she had been in months. All three were enjoying happiness once again. One year later, Daisy passed gracefully in her sleep.

Daisy's lesson to us all is to remember to be present with whatever is occurring in the moment. Be truthful. If you feel sad, then say so. Your dog already feels what you are feeling, so tell it like it is. It's OK to explain to your beloved companion that it will be hard for you when he is gone. Share that you will get through it, and that you will be OK eventually. He must hear this to know he won't be letting you down when he cannot stay to take care of you. His time inevitably will come to an end. By being honest and present today, you will empower your sweet loved one to have a peaceful transition in the future.

I urge you to celebrate the treasure of each and every day with your senior friend. Assuredly, your loyal companion is doing the same with you. Simply do your personal best to remain in a place of love rather than worry, presence rather than fear, and enjoy the magic within your dog's golden years.

Terri O' Hara has been offering her services as an Animal Communicator since 1995. She has helped thousands of people and their animal companions nationally and internationally, working with dogs, cats, horses, and many other domestic animals. Her services include intuitive consultations to assist people in understanding what animals are thinking and feeling. Terri also provides workshops, retreats, public presentations, and an apprenticeship program.

Animalwize, LLC
541-752-2020 or 800-515-9064
www.Animalwize.com
Animalwize@aol.com

My Favorite Resources:

Helping Elder Animals by Terri O'Hara,
A podcast available for download at
    www.AnimalWize.com
Learning Their Language – Intuitive Communication with Animals and Nature, by Marta Williams,
    www.MartaWilliams.com
Language of Animals – 7 Steps to Communicating with Animals, by Carol Gurney,
    www.GurneYinstitute.com
Animal Talk – Interspecies Telepathic Communication, by Penelope Smith
    www.AnimalTalk.net

Animal Voices, Animal Guides – Discovering Your Deeper Self Through Communication with Animals
by Dawn Baumann Brunke
> *www.AnimalVoices.net*

How to Communicate with Animals: Introduction to Telepathic Animal Communication, a webinar by Teresa Wagner
> *www.AnimalsInOurHearts.com*

Conversations With Animals – Cherished Messages and Memories as Told by an Animal Communication by Lydia Hiby
> *www.LydiaHiby.com*

Dogs That Know When Their Owners Are Coming Home: And Other Unexplained Powers of Animals by Rupert Sheldrake
> *www.ShelDrake.org*

Animal Communicator Directory at
> *www.AnimalTalk.net*

Animal Spirit Healing & Education Network
Internet classes, online forums, and social networking.
> *www.AnimalSpiritNetwork.com*

6

Senior Dog Nutrition Basics
with Susan Lauten, Ph.D.

Are the majority of dogs overweight?

What are some good supplements for my senior dog?

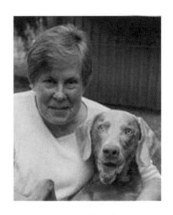

Nutritional needs can vary greatly among the different breeds of dogs. While some will weigh less than a pound at birth, others will reach an adult weight of as much as 250 pounds. A Chihuahua does not age at the same rate as a Saint Bernard and the different nutritional needs of all breeds should be taken into account. Aging causes a decrease in the functional ability of organs and these differences can vary widely between individual dogs. Generally, the larger the dog is, the shorter his expected life span will be—it would appear the dietary needs for a 10-year-old small breed dog are not the same as for a 10-year-old large breed dog. We know that a lifetime of nutrition has a definite impact on the health and wellbeing of our senior dogs. So, what can we do to help?

As with most species, aging in dogs brings a general decline in immune system function, a decline in the total number of cells and an increase in the ratio of fat to lean tissue. Some level of dehydration is also found both within cells and between cells. This fluid loss plays an important role in overall health. What we see are changes in senses such as hearing, eyesight, smell and taste. Hearing and eyesight become less acute and smell and taste are frequently diminished with increasing age. Since appetite is strongly associated with taste and smell, these changes can cause decreased food intake and play an important role in the diet of a senior dog. Interestingly, the ability to digest food doesn't appear to be significantly different for dogs through the geriatric stage.

Some important scientific discoveries made in the past 15 years have helped nutritionists better define the dietary needs of the senior dog. For instance, Purina® scientists demonstrated that monitoring food intake to maintain a lean and trim dog resulted in longer, healthier lives for those animals. Study results also indicate that dogs maintained at proper body weight show a significant delay in the onset of typical signs associated with the aging process.

> *Maintaining your furry family member at an ideal body weight is probably the most important contributor to a long and healthy life for your dog.*

Many dog families fall short of this goal. At this writing, 60 percent of dogs and cats are overweight. It is now so common to see "fat" dogs and cats that our mental picture of "healthy weight" has been altered. How does the average pet family determine if their own four-legged family member is overweight?

The best tool available to you is your hands. Whether your dog is young or old, your hands can determine whether your dog is under or overweight; how much muscle mass he has; and if his coat is thinning or his skin is dry. If you begin this process when you first bring a dog into your family, you will have very important memories in your hands and mind and you will more than likely have a longer relationship with your new family member.

- Starting at the neck, feel how round it is or isn't. Round and firm would indicate muscle mass like that of a younger dog. The shoulders should have good muscle cover, but you should still be able to palpate or feel the shoulder blades.

  - When going down from the top of the back, the spinal column should be palpable, fairly close to the skin, but not visually obvious.

  - The ribs should be easily felt through about a quarter to a half inch of skin and fat. (If your dog is short-coated, the last three ribs should be visible when the dog is trotting or running in front of you).

  - For the hips, the points of the pelvis should be palpable, one on each side of the top of the lower back. You may have to push a little to find them, but they should be able to be felt.

  - Lastly, the base of the tail can tell us about excess weight. At the point where body meets tail is a small, almost triangular area that should NOT be identifiable. I call it the dimple that we do not want to see. If it is visible, the dog is carrying excess fat on his back.

Remember: the Purina Lifetime Study proved that lean dogs have longer, healthier lives. Please be sure that the four-legged members of your family are not in the 60 percent of overweight animals.

Once you've determined your dog's weight status, you will want to adjust caloric intake accordingly.

Caloric intake or energy is provided by a combination of protein, fat and carbohydrate. If we chart caloric requirements and the weight of dog, we find that the relationship is not linear; smaller dogs require slightly more energy intake (proportionately to their size).

Some specific breeds (such as Labrador retrievers, Golden retrievers, Beagles and Dachshunds) have a tendency toward weight gain—we assume this is a genetic trait and not the result of feeding practices. Due to biologic changes such as loss of lean muscle mass and an increase in fat tissue (fat tissue is not a metabolic tissue and therefore does not require energy to function), it has been determined that energy requirements decline by approximately 20 percent in all geriatric dogs. Since there are no changes in digestive capabilities, it is assumed that the decrease in energy requirements is due to loss of muscle mass.

If your dog is overweight, the ration restriction of 20 percent to account for loss of lean muscle, as described above, is a good starting point. If sufficient weight loss is not achieved, then switching to a senior food with high quality protein and lower fat is recommended.

If your dog is not overweight, there is no physiologic need for a senior diet. A high quality, highly digestible, moderate fat diet should suffice for older dogs of healthy weight. Protein levels of 28-30 percent dry matter, fat levels of 10-14 percent dry matter and calories of about 350 per cup would represent a good diet. New legislation now requires pet foods to contain caloric contents of food on the package. Fully balanced home-cooked diets are also good choices for senior dogs as they can be formulated to meet the needs of your four-legged family member to provide the right amount of energy, with appropriate protein, fat, vitamins, minerals and antioxidants. Selection of home-cooked recipes should be limited to those that are described as fully balanced for maintenance or weight loss. A qualified nutritionist can formulate a custom diet for your dog or diets from various sources may be used. Remember, they must be balanced diets, formulated to meet the requirements of the Association of American Feed Control Officials (AAFCO).

Let's take a look at some other nutritional considerations for senior dogs:

Water: Dogs should be encouraged to drink. Water is the most important nutrient for short-term survival of an animal. In the senior dog, fluid intake should be carefully monitored, and at all times fresh, clean water should be available to dogs.

Water can also be added to food. Very diluted broths will frequently entice a dog to drink, while some dogs will eat ice cubes (Caution: there is some risk of tooth damage). There is currently no research into regulation of water intake in senior dogs, but data from human studies are deemed to be applicable to dogs. In controlled environments, older humans are able to consume adequate fluids for daily maintenance. However, when challenged by water deprivation through exercise and/or a warm environment, fluid replacement (by drinking) has been found to not be adequate in elderly humans. Consequently, the hydration status of the senior dog should be carefully monitored in warm and/or humid temperatures and during periods of exercise.

Do not assume that the dog will rehydrate himself naturally.

In addition, it's important to remember that the kidneys depend on water to perform their function of filtering waste products—if any kidney function has been lost over time, the need for fluid intake increases.

Carbohydrates: Older dogs do not experience any decline in the ability to absorb sugars and sugar alcohols, but as young dogs, they absorbed glucose more slowly than they do now. There is also evidence that insulin resistance increases with age in dogs, suggesting that our senior dogs would likely benefit from food ingredients with lower glycemic indices. Starch (a simple carbohydrate) is a major component of commercial dog diets and would have a high glycemic index. For the senior dog, substitute with more whole grains and vegetables which would represent more complex carbohydrates and lower glycemic meals.

Fat (Lipids): As dogs age, we have accepted that energy expenditure decreases which in turn reduces the animal's lean body mass while the fat mass increases. Fat is not metabolic tissue, meaning it does not require energy to maintain itself, whereas muscle requires energy to work and to remain active. Therefore, the quantity of fat in the diet of a senior dog can be safely reduced if signs of obesity are present.

Even so, there are essential fatty acids required, namely linoleic and alpha-linolenic acid. As long as the diet is formulated to meet AAFCO requirements, the essential fatty acids are included in sufficient quantities, while other fats have been limited. In 2006, the Nutritional Research Council (NRC) included a recommendation for omega-3 fatty acids in dog diets. Specifically 110 mg of EPA and DHA are recommended per 1,000 calories of food. You will now find different sources of fish oils in all dog foods. The anti-inflammatory properties of fish oils are of great benefit to the senior dog (e.g., arthritis).

Protein: Conventional wisdom previously determined that protein was detrimental to kidneys, so senior diets were formulated with less protein in an attempt to "spare" the kidneys at a time when kidney disease was associated with aging. Current knowledge suggests that senior dogs need more protein to provide building blocks for cells that are being replaced at a rate faster than those of a younger dog. In order to maintain lean tissue and immune system function senior dogs need to receive approximately 25 percent of calories from protein.

Protein needs can also be expressed as grams of protein per kilogram (1 kilogram is equal to 2.2 pounds of body weight). It has been suggested that 4.5 grams of digestible protein is required for every kilogram of body weight. This value is about 50 percent higher than that of adult dogs.

It is also important to carefully select the type of protein fed to senior dogs. Highly digestible proteins are more important to the senior dog than they are to younger dogs. The ability to digest does not change with aging, but efficiency of digestion does (slowed GI motility, alterations in enzyme activity, impaired circulation affecting absorption of nutrients).

It's important to present the digestive tract with high quality, easily digestible proteins. Minimally processed animal source proteins, such as muscle meats, offal and eggs are more easily digested than cereal proteins, meat meals, and rendered proteins from animal by-products. If the feed ingredients are not easily digestible, the body must then work to eliminate the indigestible food matter. As discussed earlier, an altered sense of smell can decrease food intake. Increased protein requirements, along with decreased intake associated with aging highlights the importance of high quality, easily digestible protein.

Minerals and Vitamins: There are specific recommendations and requirements made by the NRC and AAFCO with regard to 12 minerals (calcium, phosphorus, magnesium, sodium, potassium, chloride, iron, copper, zinc, manganese, selenium and iodine). However, few studies have been undertaken for the changes in requirements associated with the aging process. In one study, mineral absorption of calcium, phosphorus, magnesium, zinc, copper, iron, potassium and sodium did not appear to differ between one-year-old Beagles and 10-12-year-old Beagles. The importance of calcium intake is limited to the period of weaning to adult, when puppies passively absorb calcium.

Once dogs mature, regulatory hormones manage absorption and excretion of calcium in healthy dogs. Other minerals such as zinc, copper, and selenium are important in senior dogs and have been reported as mineral deficiencies more frequently than other minerals, indicating a possible increased need for these minerals.

It is also possible that intestinal absorption lessens or excretion increases during aging. Supplementing with low levels of the fat soluble vitamins A, D, E and K is suggested to counteract this development. As kidneys age, they frequently excrete the water-soluble vitamins in higher concentrations than young dogs. To compensate, supplements containing water-soluble B vitamins: B1, 2, 3, 5, 6 and 12, are suggested for these dogs. Other vitamins recommended include pantothenic acid, choline, folate and biotin. Increased levels of these vitamins are often found in commercial senior dog diets.

If you are feeding an adult maintenance diet and choose to supplement with various nutrients, look for this symbol on the pet supplements

you buy: This is the symbol for the National
Animal Supplement Council (NASC). Supplements are not regulated by the FDA, and are not
always pure, safe and effective. The NASC has
guidelines and requirements before their seal can
be affixed to a pet product.

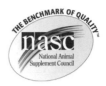

Mental Health: There is a condition in dogs that is quite similar to
Alzheimer disease in humans. The term given to the condition is Canine
Cognitive Dysfunction Syndrome (CCDS or CDS). The changes associated with CDS are specific and can be subjectively evaluated by a pet
family over time. These symptoms include:

- Disorientation (e.g. not remembering which side a door opens
  from or not knowing where the usual feeding location is);

- Changes in interactions with people or other animals (e.g., not
  recognizing people they know, an increased aggression toward
  familiar people or family members, including other animal
  family members like the family cat or a second dog);

- Sleep-wake cycle disruptions (e.g. dog paces through the house
  at night when they should be asleep);

- Loss of house breaking habits, increased or inappropriate
  vocalization; and

- Changes in activity levels (this can be an increased activity as
  well as a decreased activity level). Some of the changes described
  above can be symptomatic of an increase in anxiety levels.

The incidence of CDS increases with age and frequently the older
the dog, the more symptoms are seen and their intensity increases.
Fortunately, we now know that nutrient supplementation can slow and
actually reverse some aging signs in dogs.

The brain contains many fragile proteins, fats and nucleotides, which are candidates for physical damage. The metabolic rate of the brain is quite high (metabolism requires oxygen). The ability to repair damage is limited as is the ability to defend against damage. Aging further reduces the brain's ability to cope with potential damage as cells function less efficiently. Antioxidants are instrumental in protecting cells from future damage and repairing damage that has been done. Once cell death has occurred, it cannot be brought back, but other cells can be utilized to perform functions of lost cells.

Vitamin E is a fat soluble vitamin that protects cell membranes, while water-soluble vitamin C replenishes vitamin E to a functional state. L-carnitine and DL-α-lipoic acid both work within the cell to enhance cell efficiency and provide additional antioxidant levels within the aging cell. Other antioxidants such as flavonoids and carotenoids are found in fruits and vegetables. Medium chain triglycerides (MCTs) provide an alternative energy supply to the brain and are another source of support for brain function in the aging dog. Thorne Research® offers many antioxidants as well as vitamins and minerals for aging dogs. The addition of fresh vegetable and fruits will also provide flavonoids and other phytonutrients. However,

Onions, grapes, raisins, macadamia nuts, avocado and chocolate are toxic to dogs—please do not feed them these foods.

Supplements: Earlier in this chapter. reference was made to antioxidants as being an excellent supplement to affect a change in cognitive function. Older dogs also face problems such as arthritis, heart disease, urinary tract infections, liver problems from corticosteroid use, a more sensitive stomach and intestinal tract, etc. Supplements should be chosen carefully, preferably with the approval of your veterinarian. Although many supplements are used for their medicinal purpose, there is no regulation of the supplement industry as there is in the pharmaceutical industry. Any claims can be made without reference to proof of efficacy and any ingredients can be added to the product. It is easy to make impulse purchases based upon advertising or word of mouth, but the purchase of any supplements or nutraceuticals should be done with the help of your veterinarian.

Typical supplements for arthritic dogs include glucosamine and chondroitin sulfate, MSM, Perna Canaliculus (green-lipped mussel) fish oils and avocado and soybean unsaponifiables. All of these products are recommended for the management of arthritis, which is an inflammatory condition. As of this writing, there is no definitive research indicating the proper amounts and mixtures of each of the above-mentioned supplements to give the best results.

Although there is scientific evidence behind products from Nutra-max® and VetriScience®, the best possible mix is yet to be determined. Use a product that works for your individual dog. Another choice is to opt for stem cell harvesting and reintroduction. Although expensive, the results of this new treatment have been excellent.

Urinary tract infections seem to become more prevalent as dogs age, particularly female dogs. The sphincter that keeps urine in the body loses some of its tone, and the potential for bacterial migration increases. Some females sit on the ground to urinate, which would increase this risk. Although there is no product that can alter urine acidity enough to prevent infection, cranberry extract has been shown to provide some benefit. The key to purchasing cranberry is to choose a standardized product. This means that the concentration of the extract is held constant, while the dose or dose per capsule may change. Without standardization in supplements, there is no way to compare products.

Cranberry extract may increase urine acidity slightly, and it is also known to make the bladder wall less adhesive. Bacteria that become unable to adhere to the bladder wall can be washed away in urine.

Heart disease, although not identical to the plaque problem humans experience, can be very serious and life threatening to senior dogs. Congestive heart failure and cardiomyopathy are just two of the most common heart diseases of older dogs. CoQ10 is a supplement that is known to provide benefits to the aging heart as well as contributing to the strength of the immune system. L-carnitine and Taurine are amino acids that are heart healthy as well. Most heart supplements contain all three of these plus various herbs.

Many dogs have been given corticosteroids over the years to control any number of inflammatory conditions, including environmental allergies. Supplements such as milk thistle and SAM-e (s adenosyl methionine) are liver protective and can be used to support liver function in the event the liver has some damage or is just not functioning as it should. There are many reliable companies that offer these products.

Gastric and intestinal problems also increase as a dog ages. Foods that may have been well tolerated in younger years may no longer be tolerated. The needs of the geriatric or senior dog include high quality, highly digestible proteins as discussed earlier. The introduction of supplements themselves can have a negative effect on a sensitive gastrointestinal tract. Sometimes some flavorings or ingredients are not well tolerated; or actual allergic reactions can occur.

> *It is best to introduce any supplement gradually to determine how the dog reacts to the product.*

Lastly, enlisting the help of your veterinarian is highly recommended. Your older dog may be taking medications that do not mix with the supplements you have chosen. Even if you have carefully selected your supplements to make sure that the companies have been in business for a long time, produce high quality products and generally have a good business track record as supplements can have negative medical effects on dogs. Drug reactions can occur with many herbs and your veterinarian can guide you through these risky side effects.

The commercial pet food market does not provide consistent products to the consumer because there are no nutritional requirements established for senior or geriatric dogs. Neither the Association of American Feed Control Officials (AAFCO) nor the (NRC) provides requirements or recommendations for nutrient levels in the diets of senior dogs.

The goals of senior dog nutrition are:

1. account for size differences and rate of aging in the individual dog;

2. delay the onset of disease;

3. increase length of life; and

4. increase the quality of life.

In order to accomplish this, senior or geriatric diets need to address dog size and relative age, changes in food digestion, nutrient metabolism, storage of nutrients, and the excretion of waste. I hope that this information helps to keep your senior dog healthy through his/her golden years.

Susan Lauten, Ph.D. *earned a Masters in Agriculture with a focus on nutrition and food allergies in dogs and then earned a PhD in Biomedical Sciences from the College of Veterinary Medicine at Auburn University. Her focus was companion animal nutrition, which included a 3+ year study into the growth and development of large breed puppies. While pursuing her graduate degrees, Dr. Lauten began training dogs, working with Weimaraner rescue, and then co-founded the Auburn animal-assisted therapy group, Pets Uplifting People's Spirits (PUPS), where Susan and her dog Kizzy, worked with hospice. After graduation, she accepted a post-doctoral position at the University of Tennessee, College of Veterinary Medicine. Dr. Lauten spent almost 6 years at the Veterinary School, offering individual case nutrition to the veterinary specialists at the college. She also provided services to area veterinarians, trained veterinary students to use nutrition as part of their clinical experience, and gave veterinary specialists up-to-date nutrition recommendations for their patients.*

Pet Nutrition Consulting
865-577-0233
www.PetNutritionConsulting.com
Info@PetNutritionConsulting.com

My Favorite Resources:

Dog Quality - Helping older dogs enjoy life
> *www.DogQuality.com/blog*

The Senior Dog Blog
> *TheSeniorDogBlog.blogspot.com*

The Grey Muzzle Organization Support and Education - about the value of senior dog citizens
> *www.GreyMuzzle.org*

The Senior Dog Project Promotes adoption of senior dogs
> *www.SRDogs.com*

Selections of senior dog books
> *www.SeniorDogBooks.com*

Pet food information and ratings
> *www.DogFoodAnalysis.com*

7

The Importance of Blood Work with Fred Metzger, DVM, Diplomate ABVP

Why is it so important to monitor my dog's blood?

Can you help me understand the tests?

Senior and geriatric veterinary medicine represents the basic mission of veterinarians and veterinary technicians—detecting diseases earlier so intervention can help improve the quality of life for older dogs, cats and their owners. Complete diagnostic efforts are critical because senior pets frequently have abnormalities in multiple body systems and frequently receive long term medications for chronic diseases or conditions related to aging.

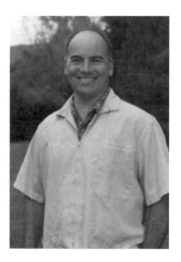

Owners are critical components to the successful senior program. Comprehensive histories are especially critical in senior medicine. Note changes in water consumption, decreased or increased appetite, alterations in body weight, decreased or increased activity level, the appearance or variations in skin masses and especially modifications in behavior. Owners are in the unique position to note subtle changes in daily routines. Behavior changes should not be discounted as "senility" without our best diagnostic efforts.

Veterinarians and their hospital team are vital components and should be vocal advocates for older patients. Older patients should receive more frequent physical examinations (twice yearly or more frequently) depending on health status, current medication history and pre-existing health problems.

Routine monitoring of blood and urine tests are important tools in the management of older patients because blood and urine testing allows the veterinarian to monitor trends in the tests which may be the earliest indicator of disease. For example, monitoring older patients for changes in blood sugar may be the earliest indicator of diabetes which is a common disease in older dogs and cats.

Defining the Senior and Geriatric Pet

The Metzger Animal Hospital Age Analogy chart which (Figure 1. on the next page) is the critical education piece for our practice's entire senior/geriatric program—it defines the senior patient. The chart graphically educates owners by showing the human age equivalent then assigns a color code or risk to the pet. For example, according to Figure 1, an 80-pound golden retriever becomes a "senior" at 6 years of age and geriatric at 10 years of age, thus emphasizing the distinction between senior and geriatric.

This classification increases client discussions and consequently diagnostic opportunities, as owners become educated about senior and geriatric diseases and our early detection recommendations including routine blood profiling on older healthy patients.

Physical, Physiological, Metabolic and Immunologic Effects of Aging

Aging affects every body system. Pet owners may recognize many of the physical changes associated with aging such as obesity, lameness and skin changes. Skin becomes thickened and less elastic and many dark

Senior Dogs

Is Your Pet A "Senior"?

You've heard that one human year equals seven dog years. Dr. Fred Metzger, DVM, developed this chart to tell you if your pet is considered a "Senior". Your veterinarian can help you to learn more about the special needs of senior and geriatric dogs and cats.

	Dog's Size (In Pounds)			
Age	0-20	21-50	51-90	>90
6	40	42	45	49
7	44	47	50	56
8	48	51	55	64
9	52	56	61	71
10	56	60	66	78
11	60	65	72	86
12	64	69	77	93
13	68	74	82	101
14	72	78	88	108
15	76	83	93	115
16	80	87	99	123
17	84	92	104	--
18	88	96	109	--
19	92	101	115	--
20	96	105	120	--

Based on a chart developed by Dr. Fred L. Metzger, DVM, Dipl. ABVP, State College, PA

Fred Metzger DVM, Diplomate ABVP
Metzger Animal Hospital

Selected biochemical profile tests commonly performed in senior dogs. The list below is for background information and is not to be used for the diagnosis of medical conditions.

coated dogs get graying of the muzzle and other areas of the coat. Muscle, bone and cartilage mass decreases. Dental tartar accumulates, calculus forms and periodontal disease occurs with resulting bad breath noticed by many owners.

Physiological effects of aging are medically very important and the kidney, liver, heart and brain are especially affected.

Aging results in a decrease in the metabolism so older pets generally require less calories. Older animals tend to have decreased activity levels resulting in increased body fat percentage. This is especially important because increased body weight results in increased incidence of diseases such as diabetes, cardiovascular, respiratory, orthopedic diseases and perhaps cancer.

Aging is also associated with an increased incidence of auto-immune or immune-mediated diseases where the body attacks itself.

Pharmacological Effects of Aging

Senior patients frequently require pharmacologic intervention for disease management. Aging affects the absorption, distribution, bio-transformation and elimination of most drugs; consequently, seniors have special medication concerns. Drug dosages may need adjusted for seniors and many drugs avoided if organ function is compromised. Pharmaceuticals eliminated by the liver and kidneys cause special concerns.

Pharmaceuticals with special concerns in geriatric patients include: antibiotics, NSAIDs, steroids, barbitutes, sedatives, analgesics, diuretics, ACE inhibitors, digitalis derivatives, chemotherapeutics, hormonal drugs, anesthetics and many others.

Routine blood profiling increases the safety of drug administration by identifying underlying disease conditions which may preclude the use of certain pharmaceuticals.

The Senior Screening Panel

The minimum senior canine panel should include the Complete Blood Count (CBC), organ function profile (biochemical profile), electrolytes (sodium, potassium, chloride), and complete urinalysis plus heartworm and tick borne disease testing in appropriate patients.

Veterinarians may elect to include an electrocardiography (ECG), blood pressure measurement and eye pressure screening for glaucoma (ocular tonometry). Fecal examination should be considered in appropriate patients especially outside dogs or cats.

Albumin: (ALB)

Albumin is produced exclusively in the liver. It is a serum protein that affects the osmotic pressure, binds calcium and transports fatty acids and many drugs.

Increased Albumin:
> Suggests dehydration

Decreased Albumin:
> Suggests starvation, parasitism, chronic malabsorptive disease, chronic liver disease, protein losing enteropathy and glomerulonephritis.

Alkaline Phosphatase (ALKP)

Alkaline phosphatase has 6 isoenzymes with liver and bone being the major isoenzymes. Elevated ALKP activity in the serum indicates increased production in the liver, bile ducts and growing bone or decreased excretion in bile and urine. The enzyme is induced by abnormally low bile flow and corticosteroid use. Because of this, ALKP is a less specific liver test.

Increased ALKP:
> Suggests liver disease caused by failure of bile flow (cholestasis), steroid use, and bone growth. ALKP can increase with pancreatitis and is commonly increased with canine Cushing's disease.

Decreased ALKP:
> Not associated with common medical conditions

Alanine Transferase (ALT)

ALT is liver specific and is released when the individual liver cells become damaged. ALT is present in large quantities in the cytoplasm of canine and feline liver cells (HEPATOCYTES). This enzyme enters the blood stream when liver cells are damaged or destroyed and circulates for a few days.

Increased ALT:

Suggests hepatocellular leakage. THIS TEST IS VERY SENSITIVE AND SPECIFIC FOR LIVER DISEASE, but does not indicate cause or reversibility of the damage.

Decreased ALT:

Not associated with common medical conditions.

Calcium

Calcium levels in extracellular fluid and bone are controlled mainly by the parathyroid hormone (PTH) and vitamin D and the interaction of these with the gut, bone, kidney and parathyroid glands.

Increased Calcium (Hypercalcemia):

Dissolving bone lesions sometimes associated with reabsorption
Hyperparathyroidism
Increased Vitamin D levels (Hypervitaminosis D)
**Malignant (cancerous) tumor of the lymphoid tissue (Lymphosarcoma) ** MOST COMMON CAUSE
Anal gland tumors
Addison's Disease (Hypoadrenocorticism)
Kidney Failure

Decreased Calcium (Hypocalcaemia):

Ethylene glycol poisoning
Pancreatitis
Low albumin levels (Hypoalbumnemia)
Vitamin D deficiency

Cholesterol (CHOL)

Cholesterol is not a diagnostic test when used alone but supplements other tests. Cholesterol is primarily produced in the liver and excreted in bile.

Increased Cholesterol:
Hypothyroidism
Obstructive biliary disease
Cushing's disease
A condition of the kidneys marked by water retention between the tissues, excessive protein in the urine, low albumin levels and elevated cholesterol levels. (Nephrotic Syndrome)

Creatinine

Creatinine is nitrogenous product of muscle metabolism. Creatinine levels are kidney specific and not as affected by diet and protein catabolism than BUN levels.

Increased Creatinine Levels:
Accumulation of constituents in the blood that are normally excreted in the urine. Can result in a severely toxic condition and can occur in severe kidney disease (UREMIA)

Glucose (GLU)

Increased Blood Glucose:
Persistent elevated levels indicate diabetes mellitus
Sample collection after eating may alter results

Decreased Blood Glucose: GLUCOSE
Insulinoma
Starvation
Addison's disease

Hypopituitarism
Shock
Severe exertion

Phosphorus (PHOS)

Control of phosphorus is complex and is influenced by the actions of PTH and vitamin D and the interaction of these hormones with the gut, bones, kidneys and parathyroid glands.

Increased PHOS:
Hemolysis (Red blood cells contain significant amounts of PHOS, hemolysis of blood samples or delayed removal of the serum from the clot can falsely elevate PHOS values.)

Renal disease (Because of the decreased amounts of PHOS being excreted in urine.)

Hypoparathyroidism

Decreased PHOS:
Hypoparathyroidism
Diabetic Ketoacidosis

Total Bilirubin (TBIL)

Bilirubin is derived from the break down of hemoglobin and circulates in conjugated and unconjugated forms. TBIL measurements are the combination of both forms.

Increased Tbili
Liver disease
Hemolytic disease (Destruction of red blood cells.)

Urea Nitrogen (BUN)

Urea is the primary solid component of urine and the end product of protein decomposition.

Increased BUN:
    Increased levels of nitrogenous waste products (Azotemia)
    Gastrointestinal hemorrhage
    Renal Disease (pre, renal or post)
    Heart disease
    Hypoadrenocorticism (Addison's Disease)
    Dehydration
    Shock

Decreased BUN:
    Porto systemic Shunt
    Severe Liver Failure

Total Protein (TP)

Total protein is the sum of the albumin and globulin in the blood. When measured on serum it usually consists of albumin, globulins and fibrinogen. It is often used as an indicator of hydration status.

Elevated TP:
    Dehydration
    Anything increasing Albumin or Globulin

Decreased TP:
    Anything decreasing Albumin or Globulin

Globulin

Globulin is primarily produced in the liver. It aids with nutritive functions and helps maintain colloidal osmotic pressure along with forming enzymes, antibodies, coagulation factors, and transport substances.

Increased Globulin:
 Chronic inflammatory disease
 Parasitism
 Neoplasia
 Immune-mediated disease

Decreased Globulin:
 Not a medical condition

Gamma Glutamyl Transpeptidase (GGT)

GGT is involved in the metabolism of a peptide called glutathione and is mainly associated with the membranes of liver cell surfaces, bile duct epithelium and renal convoluted tubular epithelial cells.

Increased GGT:
 Cholestatic liver disease
 Cushing's disease
 Disease of the portal biliary system

Decreased GGT:
 Not clinically significant

Lipase (LIPA)

Lipase is the primary enzyme responsible for the decomposition of fat.

Increased Lipase:
 Pancreatitis (acute and chronic)
 Renal failure
 Intestinal inflammation
 Small intestinal obstruction
 Following the administration of steroids
 GI perforation

Decreased Lipase:
   Not clinically significant

Summary-Senior Health Program Benefits

Earlier detection allows earlier intervention and therefore, improved treatment success. Senior profiling improves anesthetic safety by identifying hidden existing diseases and permitting the postponement of anesthesia or altering the anesthetic plan. Furthermore, pharmaceutical safety is increased through detection of underlying diseases, which may preclude the use of certain drugs or suggest new alternative treatments.

Many dietary recommendations are based on disease diagnosis making senior profiling an important dietary database. Finally, earlier disease management by improved anesthetic, pharmaceutical and dietary recommendations offer our patient's and client's the best medical management possible.

Dr. Fred Metzger is a 1986 graduate of the Purdue School of Veterinary Medicine and a Diplomate of the American Board of Veterinary Practitioners (Canine/Feline). He is an Adjunct Professor at Penn State University and serves on the practitioner advisory boards of Veterinary Economics and Veterinary Medicine magazines. Dr. Metzger owns the Metzger Animal Hospital, a six -doctor general and referral practice in State College, Pennsylvania.

Metzger Animal Hospital
1044 Benner Pike
State College, PA 16801
814-237-5333
FLMDVM@aol.com
www.MetzgerAnimal.com

My Favorite Resources:

Idexx Laboratories
Continuing education for veterinary practitioners,technicians
and managing professionals.
www.IdexxLearningCenter.com

Veterinary Partner
Support for you and your veterinarian in the care of dogs with
up to the date animal health information.
www.VeterinaryPartner.com

Vet Information
Blood and lymph disorders in dogs
www.VetInfo.com

Terrific Pets.com
www.TerrificPets.com

Blood disorder information
Info Vets
Condition and Diseases Info.
www.InfoPets.com

Senior Dog Resources
www.SrDogs.com

Dog Blog and Information
www.AllThingsDogsBlog.com

8

Senior Dog Dental Care
with Maia Bazjanac, ADH

How important is dental care for my senior dog?

I have never brushed my dog's teeth, how do I do it?

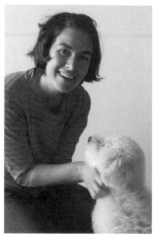

It's hard to think of another health condition that is as prevalent in older dogs as periodontal disease. When you add in broken or injured teeth, abscesses, gingival hyperplasia (overgrowth of gum) and oral cancer, oral health problems in older dogs are ubiquitous. In fact, it is actually quite unusual to find an older dog that does not have oral health issues. Even dogs that have had naturally good teeth throughout their lives almost always have some kind of decline in oral health in old age.

Unfortunately, poor oral health significantly decreases the quality of life for an elderly dog and can even shorten his life in more ways than you might expect.

The basics of caring for your older dog's dental health are really very straightforward. First, you'll need to determine whether your dog has any conditions in his mouth that require immediate medical attention. These would most commonly include periodontal (gum) disease and loose or broken teeth. I recommend an oral examination by a veterinarian who will evaluate your pet's mouth for any current or potential issues.

If this examination reveals that your dog has any obvious signs of gum disease, including recessed gums, swollen or bleeding gums, or even just bad breath, she should have a veterinary dental cleaning done under anesthesia. If any teeth need extraction, this will also require anesthesia. If your dog has healthy gums and no other oral health issues, but still needs calculus removed, you may be able to have it done without anesthesia. However, this is an option that is only appropriate if it is very clear your dog has no oral health problems, so it's important not to be too attached to having it done this way. Making sure that any potential medical issues are accurately assessed is essential, and sometimes this cannot be done without anesthesia.

The thought of anesthesia is upsetting for some pet owners, as many people fear their pet may either die while under anesthesia or experience bad health consequences as a result of anesthesia. While these fears are not irrational, per se, they are generally not in proportion to the realistic outcomes associated with anesthesia. While there is always a risk of complications (including, rarely, death), I can absolutely guarantee you that dogs are much more likely to have significant health issues as a result of gum disease than they are as a result of anesthesia. So, if your dog needs a dental procedure involving anesthetic and your vet feels it is safe, please do not avoid or even delay having it done.

In many cases, problems in the mouth exacerbate an animal's poor health, and getting the mouth cleaned up can make a big difference in improving your pet's overall well-being.

Of course, each animal needs to be evaluated individually for his or her anesthetic risks, particularly older dogs that are in poor health. Thankfully, it has become a relatively safe process in modern veterinary medicine. In general, anesthesia should not be feared. It is an amazing medical tool which allows your pet to undergo necessary and beneficial procedures with very little pain.

As an aside, it is important to note that veterinary dentistry is a relatively new discipline, and some vets have not updated their practices to include modern dental procedures. Unfortunately, these procedures can be quite expensive, but, frankly, if you are going to spend money to put your dog under anesthesia for dental work, you should get as many of the benefits as possible.

Make sure your vet is up-to-date on dental procedures and that they or a certified veterinarian technician, with current dental training, will be doing the cleaning.

Brushing Always Works

Once your veterinarian addresses any immediate oral health issues, you are ready to start doing home care. Home care is the most important aspect of your dog's oral hygiene. Getting a dog's teeth professionally cleaned does not usually "fix" all the problems. Gum disease, in particular, is a chronic condition with no cure. Regular, thorough brushing will do a lot to slow down the disease, and in some cases even stop it from progressing. If your older dog does not have gum disease, count your blessings ... and then start brushing daily to ensure that he never does!

I know, I know. You're thinking, "Do I really have to brush my dog's teeth? I can barely take care of my own teeth." I hear this a lot. Brushing your dog's teeth can seem like a chore, especially if your dog isn't particularly cooperative. But, here's the thing: it works. In fact, it is really the only thing that *always* works.

There are other things that work for some dogs sometimes, such as chewing on bones, or getting regular dental cleanings. But the only thing I know of that will always improve the health of the gums is daily brushing. Please don't misunderstand this to mean that you should skip getting your dog's teeth professionally cleaned; you shouldn't. Just understand that gum disease is caused by the daily onslaught of bacteria under the gum-line, so periodic removal of calculus can only do so much to prevent it. (Imagine what would happen in your mouth if you didn't brush your teeth and just went to the dentist once a year for a cleaning.)

True, even with regular brushing—just as with humans—some dogs will still develop gum disease (just as some people do, even with good hygiene practices). However, brushing makes a huge difference, and based on my experience, it seems to do a lot more than any single other thing to stop gum disease from developing. Because it stimulates the gums and removes bacteria on a daily basis, it can prevent gum disease in dogs with good oral health and it can dramatically slow the progression of disease in dogs that already have oral health problems.

Brushing your dog's teeth is actually quite easy, even if your dog hates it and resists your efforts. With a few tricks, just about anyone should be able to do a decent job of brushing. Here are simple instructions for brushing. But don't feel obligated to do it exactly like this. If you find a way that works better for your dog, by all means, use it. Whatever is easiest for you and your dog is the best method.

Brushing Teeth for Bigger Dogs

Standing, straddle your dog from behind, facing the same direction as he is. Hold his muzzle, so that you are holding his mouth shut. Your grip should be gentle but firm enough to let him know you want him to hold still. Point the toothbrush head towards you; slide it inside the dog's cheek on one side, and go all the way to the back. Brush in circular motions so that you are brushing the teeth and the lower and upper gum, as well. Count to ten while you brush all of the molars and premolars. Then slide the brush forward and brush the upper and lower canine teeth (the large "fangs").

Again, make sure you brush the gums, too. Count to five while you do this. Brush the very front teeth and gum-line, counting to five while you do this, as well. Do the canines on the other side, counting to five. Finish off by doing the premolars and molars on the second side, making sure you push as far back as you can so that you don't miss the back teeth. Count to ten as you do this. If you've been keeping count, that whole process should take about 35 seconds.

Unless your dog has significant gum problems, don't worry about brushing the lingual surfaces (those directly facing the tongue). (See "special circumstances" section below for instructions on brushing lingual surfaces.) Brush every day.

Brushing Teeth for Smaller Dogs

You do this almost exactly the way you would with a larger dog, except that you kneel instead of stand. Have your dog sit. Kneeling, straddle her from behind, facing the same direction as she is. Keep your feet together behind her, so she doesn't back out between your legs. Hold her muzzle firmly and gently, so that you are holding her mouth shut. Now follow the instructions above, as described for a larger dog.

Special Circumstances

"Difficult" dogs

Some dogs offer strong resistance to having their teeth brushed. There are two schools of thought on this issue. Many people advocate using flavored toothpaste to entice the dog. This way, the owner slowly "sneaks" the brushing in as the dog eats the toothpaste, rather than forcefully "imposing" it. This is a valid approach, and if you feel this is the best route for your dog, use it. If your dog is fearful and easily spooked, this would be a good way to begin so that your dog learns to associate brushing with something positive.

However, I find that in a majority of cases, resistance is a behavioral issue, exacerbated by a certain dynamic between owner and dog. I say this because, in most of these cases where an owner can't seem to get the dog to cooperate initially, I have no problem at all brushing the dog's teeth with my usual method. Generally, all it takes to resolve this issue is owners learning to hold their dogs properly, so that they have more confidence and don't end up ceding to their dogs' resistance. Dogs quickly learn to cooperate.

I don't advocate my method out of some need to insist that people have a specific dynamic with their pets. Mainly, I prefer it over the "flavored toothpaste" approach because people rarely manage to do a good job brushing with that method. While a small percentage of dogs just will not tolerate brushing, please do not assume that your dog falls into that category simply because he or she resists initially. I tell my clients to have the attitude of a "mama dog" that is doing necessary grooming for her pup. If your dog dislikes brushing, remember that the benefits of brushing are enormous and well worth a small, daily unpleasantness—35 seconds worth. Your dog will learn to deal with it, I promise.

Brushing Lingual Surfaces of the Teeth

Some dogs build up tartar very quickly. In these cases, the benefits of trying to brush the inside surfaces of their teeth outweigh the downside (which is that it is quite difficult to do well, and it can make the whole brushing process a bit more stressful).

For these dogs, I recommend that you start by bushing the facial (facing outward) surfaces and acclimate your dog to that before adding the lingual surfaces to the process. Once you and your dog have gotten pretty good at the facial surfaces, you can step up the brushing to include the lingual surfaces.

To do this, you will still hold your dog's mouth shut, but with enough slack in your hand that your dog can slightly open her jaw.

Slide the toothbrush inside the mouth just behind the canine teeth. Point it towards the throat to do the back teeth, and then point it forward to do the inside of the canines and the incisors. This may take a little practice. Your dog may resist this more than she does brushing the facial surfaces, simply because it's more disturbing for her to feel as if something is being shoved so far inside her mouth. Just be calm, gentle and firm, and keep it short and sweet. No need to overdo it in the beginning. As you do it more and more, your dog will get used to it, and you'll get better at it yourself.

Other Important Tips for Home Care

The one thing I want to stress is that brushing should be done every day. It takes about 24-48 hours for the plaque on teeth to start calcifying. Ideally, you want to remove the plaque (which is a slimy filmy substance) before this happens, as once it calcifies (and turns into hard tarter) it is much harder to remove. So, brushing every day is actually significant.

I generally recommend brushing right before you feed your dog. This serves two purposes. First, your dog will begin to associate brushing with getting fed, which is a positive thing. Second, you will be less likely to forget to brush if you attach it to feeding—since, hypothetically at least, you won't forget to feed your dog!

If you have a dog that isn't particularly food-motivated, or who doesn't get fed on a regular schedule, this may be a little less effective for you. In that case, I'd recommend picking any time that will be easy to remember: for example, right after your morning walk, or right before bedtime. Making it a daily routine is the key to staying consistent.

I have mixed feelings regarding toothpaste and other pet dental products. Most dog toothpastes have enzymes in them and claim to inhibit the growth of plaque, but the research I've seen doesn't prove that there is any more benefit to brushing with the toothpaste than without, and the list of ingredients in toothpastes aren't that healthy.

Dogs don't rinse and spit like we do, after all, and so, end up swallowing the toothpaste.

But more significantly, many people report that using flavored toothpastes actually makes brushing much harder to do effectively because their dogs try to chew or lick the brush the whole time they are brushing. The only real benefit I see to flavored toothpaste is that it makes brushing a positive experience for a dog, but I think this can be accomplished just as well by giving your dog a treat (or simply feeding him) after brushing. However, as I said before, flavored toothpastes can be helpful with skittish or fearful dogs.

If your dog has advanced gum disease, he might benefit from some kind of oral mouthwash that kills bacteria in the mouth. Veterinary products with Chlorhexidine in them work quite well. Remember, dogs don't rinse and spit—if your dog has any serious digestive issues, these products may not be appropriate. You should consult your vet before using any.

There are also many products for gum disease that can be added to food or water, some of which seem to work better than others. I won't recommend any specifically, because I find that each animal is different. Some of these products seem to do wonders for one dog and nothing at all for another. Feel free to try them if you like, but remember that nothing will eliminate the need to brush. Ultimately, it's the mechanical act of brushing that does the most good. Even if you chose to wet your dog's brush with water and just brush with that, your dog would benefit much more than from any product you bought to replace brushing.

One of the greatest things about providing good oral hygiene for your old dog is that he won't have stinky breath. That makes it all the more wonderful to hug and kiss him every day, something which is a benefit to you both.

Good oral health is truly a boon for your elderly dog. Make it a priority in his life and let your dog live out his last years with comfort and grace.

Maia Bazjanac is a graduate of UC Berkeley and has lived in the Bay Area of Northern California since 1988. She has worked as an anesthesia-free dental hygienist for dogs and cats since 2001 and has cleaned literally thousands of animals' teeth. Over the years, in consultation with vets and human dental professionals, Maia has developed a practice that focuses on educating pet-owners, teaching easy and manageable home-care routines, and helping pet-owners set realistic long-term goals for their pet's dental health. She is known not only for her ability to communicate with her furry clients, but also for her ability to motivate and empower pet-owners to take charge of their pet's oral health.

Maia Bazjanac
510-882-8255
www.PetTooth.com
Maia@PetTooth.com

My Favorite Resources:

Pet health information
  www.Dogs.About.com
UC Davis Medical School
  www.VetmMed.UCDavis.edu
American Veterinarian Dental College
  www.AVDC.org
Dog Blog
  www.BlogPaws.com

Dog News and Resources
www.ILoveDogs.com
National List of Available Dogs for Adoption
www.SafeHarbor.com

9

Physical Therapy for the Senior Dog with Martha Pease, PT, CCRP

What is a "Biomechanics Specialist" and how can they help my dog?

Can Hydrotherapy help with my dog's arthritis?

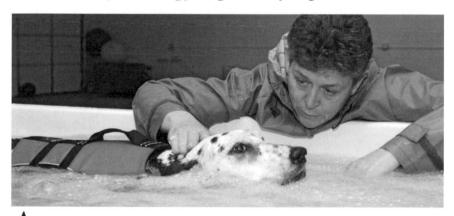

As a dog gets older and a little stiffer when getting up and moving around, owners often start to wonder what options exist to help their pet. **Physical therapy**, also called "**canine rehabilitation**," is one way to help older dogs stay active and mobile. Any human condition helped by physical therapy also applies to dogs. The approach is different, but the principles are very much the same.

For the geriatric dog, physical therapy goals include pain control, maintaining range of motion and flexibility and maintaining or improving strength, therefore helping the dog stay as active as possible. When a dog experiences less pain, he is better able to climb stairs, get up from the floor or jump on the couch. A therapist's overall goal is to improve the animal's ability to maneuver in the house, participate in sporting activities, position to urinate and defecate, go for a walk and function in other ways. With physical therapy, the dog may live longer and have an improved quality of life in its later years.

Before the dog sees a canine rehabilitation practitioner, it is very important that a veterinarian examine the pet to rule out and/or treat other possible medical conditions. Some health issues, such as infection or cancer, can mimic musculoskeletal problems.

Physical therapists are **biomechanics specialists**. They assess the musculoskeletal and nervous systems for any issues that might be contributing to the dog's functional difficulties. The evaluation is the pivotal step in determining the dog's rehabilitation activities and assessing subsequent improvements and changes. The evaluation consists of: getting medical information from the veterinarian; obtaining the dog's history from the owner; observing the dog's mobility and gait; assessing the animal's range of motion, strength and neurological deficits, and palpating to discover areas of pain, tenderness, tightness, muscle atrophy and swelling.

The dog's history is very important, particularly for the senior animal.

How long has the problem been going on? The answer to this helps determine if the condition is acute or chronic and enables the practitioner to make a prognosis for the extent of recovery.

What has the owner observed regarding the problem? He or she might mention the dog's difficulty getting up the stairs; the dog may be either hesitant, walks with bunny hops, needs momentum or requires help. This gives a picture of the extent of the dog's weakness and creates milestones by which to measure progress.

Another very important piece of information is how the owner perceives pain in the dog.

Does the dog hide more?

Avoid playing with other dogs?

Become grumpy with other dogs?

Has the dog stopped greeting the owner at the door?

These are all indications that a dog is in distress.

In the next portion of the evaluation, the practitioner will observe how the dog moves. For example,

Does the dog struggle to get up, using mostly the front legs?

Is the dog limping?

Is the animal's coordination abnormal?

Does the dog stand comfortably or is all the weight on the front legs?

Or does it pick up a leg?

These can be indications of pain or weakness. Limping can be from discomfort or weakness and lack of trust in the leg. Using front legs to get up or shifting weight forward is indicative of rear leg pain or lack of strength. Impaired coordination usually implies an underlying neurological problem. After this, the hands-on examination begins.

What is the quality of the muscling?

Is there muscle atrophy?

Is there tenderness?

Do some of the joints feel thickened, have palpable boney changes
*   or seem tender or swollen?*

What is the range of motion of each joint?

Is there any ligamentous laxity?

Ligaments are like leather straps that hold the bones in place. If they are injured or stretched out, there is too much wiggle in the join. The therapist will also assess the spine for flexibility and joint mobility of the vertebra as well as tenderness along the spinal muscles. The practitioner will also test the dog's reflexes to see if they indicate any neurological abnormalities.

After the practitioner thoroughly examines the dog, all the information from the veterinarian, the owner and the physical examination are put together to determine the main problem within the musculoskeletal system that is affecting the dog's ability to move and function. A treatment plan is designed to meet that dog's needs and will include instruction for both home and in-clinic care.

A home exercise program may include light massage, gentle stretches and range-of-motion exercises for joint health, and simple strengthening exercises. Often, a very important component of the home program is leash walks. Regular walks, even if they are very short, are critical. The older dog often is less active and, therefore, gets weaker. This becomes a vicious cycle. Walks encourage the dog to move and help maintain strength. Daily outings keep the dog mentally engaged, especially if the dog enjoys walks. Regular exercise is beneficial for organ health, as well.

In the clinic, treatment varies based on what equipment each clinic has and what that practitioner has found the most helpful. In-clinic treatments may include massage, stretching, cold laser, ultrasound, electrical stimulation, acupuncture, strength and coordination exercises, and hydrotherapy.

Hydrotherapy

Hydrotherapy includes exercise on an underwater treadmill, as well as swimming, and is particularly helpful. It has many benefits for all dogs, but can have an especially dramatic effect on senior dogs, providing a painless, fun means of exercise and movement. The relief it offers can carry over for several days, and many owners even credit hydrotherapy for extending their pet's life.

Dulci, for example, was a thirteen-year-old Wheaten terrier with spondylosis who had lost the spring in her step. Spondylosis is arthritic and boney changes along the spine that can cause stiffness and if severe, can encroach on the nerves and cause neurological problems. The last two years of her life, she received laser to her spine, as well as exercise in an underwater treadmill. Dulci's owners felt the hydrotherapy added a year to her life and improved the quality of those years, as well.

Travis was an arthritic Australian Shepherd whose elbows were very, very stiff. It was extremely painful for him to walk. Swimming was the one exercise he could do without pain. Again, the owner felt the aquatic exercise kept him around an additional two years.

Jake was a 90+ pound Great Dane/Lab mix who was weak in the rear and, for this reason, was having more and more trouble getting up from the floor and climbing stairs. The owner walked him every day, but he still needed more exercise. At first, Jake swam twice a month, but as he got older, he needed the exercise once a week. If he didn't swim, the owner noticed he would again struggle to climb stairs and rise from the floor. Being a big dog, it was important that he could do these things without much help. Hydrotherapy proved invaluable to his health as he aged.

Why does hydrotherapy work so well? The reason is relatively simple: The water provides buoyancy, which diminishes the stress on the joints, allowing the dog to move without pain. Also, the dog moves his legs in a different manner than walking during treatment, which results in more range of motion and stretching of the joints and muscles. The water also offers resistance for muscle strengthening.

Swimming

Swimming takes all the weight off of the joints, which is very helpful for arthritic dogs in particular. The uncompressed movement stimulates the joint lubricants, and the gentle range of motion that occurs during swimming decreases pain. Older dogs are commonly arthritic in their elbows and wrists and swimming helps increase the range of motion of those joints. During the swimming stroke, the animal's hocks and stifles in the rear legs are used through the full range of motion which doesn't occur with walking.

Swimming is a great means of strengthening the body because of the water resistance. It's a significant bonus to the dog. While swimming, dogs use their front legs more than the rear, which builds up muscles in the shoulders. But the rear legs also get exercised, which is important for arthritic hips. While immersed in water, the dog also works the trunk muscles abdominals and paraspinale muscles to keep the body stable. For the dog with back or neurological problems, trunk strength is key to its ability to get around.

For the weak or the neurologically impaired dog that can't support itself against gravity, water exercise is liberating. With swimming, the dog can move without falling or having to hold himself up. Its muscles are used differently than on land, which can help with coordination and cross training. Cross training is helpful because the muscles are used in a different way than on land which helps with neuromuscular retaining and stretching soft tissues. While in the water, the practitioner can stimulate movement and work with patterning to retrain correct limb usage.

The Underwater Treadmill

For dogs that are uncomfortable having their feet off the ground, swimming may be a problem. In this case, the underwater treadmill is a nice alternative. For some specific conditions, such as tibial plateau leveling osteotomies, bicipital tendonitis or neck problems, the treadmill is the hydrotherapy equipment of choice.

With this exercise, the dog is placed in the treadmill while it is empty. The water then comes up around the animal. Most of the underwater treadmills are contained in a dog run size container either made of glass or Plexiglas and the treadmill itself forms the bottom of the box. The water height is adjusted to the individual dog. The higher the water, the more the reduction of compression forces on the dog's joints.

When the water is at hip level, weight bearing is reduced by 60 percent. This is very helpful for arthritic or weak dogs. When the water is at shoulder height, dogs tend to prance. As a result, they move their joints through a broader range of motion than they do by walking. Increasing the water to hock height makes the dog pick up its legs even more, which is helpful to increase the stifle range of motion.

The neurologically impaired dog may have active movement of its legs but not enough strength to support itself against gravity. In this case, the water height can be set to the point where the body weight is supported enough for the dog to walk but low enough that the dog is still challenged.

Anyone who has been on a treadmill knows that if they don't focus and keep up with the treadmill, there will be problems. The same is true for dogs. They react to the movement under their feet by walking and quickly understand that they have to keep up with the treadmill. This improves coordination. In addition, when the dog is walking in place, the practitioner is able to manually assist with leg movement and patterning as needed.

Manual Therapy

At times, manual therapy and stretching and strengthening exercises are done in the water. The water assists with stretching exercises by helping to float the limb. On land, the dog may be too weak or in too much pain to take full weight onto a limb whereas with the body supported by the water, the dog is able to support itself on two or three legs to begin early strengthening. Having the dog go from sit to stand is like doing a squat at the gym. The dog may not be able to do this out of the water because of weakness. In the water, the buoyancy of the water aids the dog to get up from sitting. These exercises can progress to land as the dog gets stronger. Massage techniques are also enhanced when done under water.

Hydrotherapy is very helpful in weight loss. To lose weight, the dog has to burn more calories than he or she takes in. But often, the older, overweight dog has trouble getting up and moving, not only because of the weight but also due to other issues, such as arthritis and heat intolerance. Therefore, exercise without the support of water is very painful. Swimming or the underwater treadmill provides body support, resistance to the muscles for strengthening and a cool environment so the dog doesn't overheat. In this way, the dog has an opportunity to exercise to burn off calories. The dog may not only lose pounds but also size and girth as the fat is converted to muscle.

Arthritis is another condition that greatly benefits from water exercise. Maintaining the range of motion of the joints is important to reduce abnormal stress on the cartilage and ligaments and hopefully prevent further joint degradation. In addition, gentle range of motion which are movements done in the middle of the available range, are very helpful to reduce pain and swelling. Strength is crucial. If the dog is strong enough to get up easily, he or she is not straining support structures such as ligaments or putting abnormal torques on the cartilage and joint surfaces, causing further degradation of the joint. Water therapy strengthens muscles and reduces stress on the joints.

All dogs exercising in water need to be carefully monitored for overexertion. This is particularly true for the senior dog. A dog's general conditioning and endurance is often diminished at this time in its life. Due to other possible medical conditions, the dog may be less tolerant of physical exertion. Breathing patterns, color of gums and tongue and signs of fatigue must be observed during the session.

Many owners are hesitant to bring their dogs to physical therapy/ hydrotherapy because their animals "don't like water." Owners need to understand that because the therapy environment is so different from anything the dog has previously experienced, the dog's response to hydrotherapy does not correlate to previous reactions it has had to baths or sprinklers. The only way to find out if a dog will enjoy or tolerate hydrotherapy is to try it. Dogs who don't like to swim or have their feet off the ground often do very well in the underwater treadmill.

The pace of hydrotherapy sessions progress is based on the dogs' reactions during each session and the animal's recovery time after he gets home. Taking a good nap at home after a therapy session is great, but the dog shouldn't still be fatigued the next day. Ideally, animals will show no signs of increased soreness or stiffness, usually noted by more limping or slowness getting up. Each session time is increased in small increments based on practitioner assessment and owner report. The dog's progress is then noted over time.

Is the dog happier (indicating less pain)?
Can the dog walk farther?
Is the dog able to get up from the floor?
Does the dog still need help getting up the stairs?
Is the dog getting onto the bed?

Physical therapy for older dogs is often an ongoing program. Regular sessions help maintain the dog's status. The frequency of the sessions depends on the effectiveness of the program and the practitioner's preference.

In summation, physical therapy and hydrotherapy in particular, has been shown to benefit older dogs. The overall result is improved quality of life and often a longer life, as well.

Martha C. Pease, PT, CCRP was Managing Partner at Canine & Conditioning Rehabilitation Group in Colorado. She received her physical therapy Masters from Columbia University in 1982 and worked for over 20 years as a human physical therapist. In 1999, she began treating dogs and is one of the first to receive the certification in canine rehabilitation from the University of Tennessee. Ms. Pease was recognized by the American Physical Therapy Association as an orthopedic clinical specialist. She has also instructed seminars on aquatic therapy for the Canine Rehabilitation Institute and AHHA.

Canine & Conditioning Rehabilitation Group
3760 S Lipan Street
Englewood, Co 80110
303-762-SWIM
www.Dog-Swim.com
McConlogue@msn.com

My Favorite Resources:

Slippery floors:

> Runners and throw rugs that have nonskid Backing, booties
> for traction.
> Mats, plastic and fabric runners
> Furniture, steps and ramps
> > *www.ConsolidatedPlastics.com*

Harness:

> Help'Em Up/ Blue Dog: has a chest and
> rear harness that can be left on the dog.
> > *www.HelpemUp.com*

Slings:

> There are a variety of slings made to support the dog under the
> belly and rear legs. A bath towel works well if the problem is
> temporary. Walk About is a sling that the dog's legs go through
> and it can be left on the dog.
> Ginger Lead is a sling and leash combination
> > *www.HandicappedPets.com*
> > *www.GingerLead.com*

Boots:

> Ruffwear has a variety of boots.
> Pawz: lightweight rubber booties for skidding and protection
> against cold, they are good for weak dogs who don't have the
> strength to advance their legs easily, they can't be left on all day

because they don't allow the paws to breathe

www.RuffWear.com

www.PawzDogBoots.com

Wheelchairs:

Doggon Wheels

www.Doggon.com

K9Karts

www.K-9carts.com

Eddies Wheels

www.EddiesWheels.com

Walkin' Wheels

www.WalkinWheels.com

Handicapped Pets:

A resource for a variety of equipment and assistive devices

www.HandicappedPets.com

Supportive braces and wraps:

Custom made braces:

www.OrthoPets.com

Wraps and braces:

www.DogLeggs.com

Wraps and braces:

www.TheraPaws.com

10

Canine Massage
and Bodywork Options
with Jennifer Kachnic, CCMT, CRP

*What different types of bodywork options are available
for my dog?*

Can it actually assist with the immune system?

Touch. Dogs love it. They thrive when they are touched. No wonder when touch is applied in a therapeutic way—commonly called "bodywork"—it can help senior dogs enormously. Bodywork improves circulation, stimulates the immune system, promotes physical and mental relaxation, alleviates depression and reduces stress (yes, dogs have stress, too; chronic pain wears on them and changes in their environment, particularly with senior dogs, can cause great anxiety). All of these contribute to the dog's healing and bring nourishment to the dog's body while flushing out

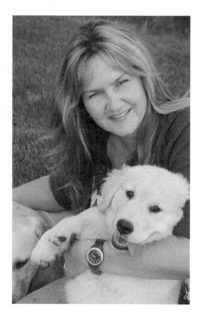

toxins. Bodywork can also break down adhesions in the dog's body, allowing damaged muscles to heal and improve range of motion.

One of the most common forms of bodywork therapy is massage. It's no surprise this is so popular. After all, who doesn't love a massage? When done correctly, massage not only feels good, but it leaves the body relaxed and gives an overall sense of well-being.

The earliest accounts of massage date back to China, 3000 B.C. It was much later, though, during the second century B.C., that Chinese medicine took the basic form it has today and practitioners began using massage as a treatment for illness. Through the years, the Chinese have developed an in-depth system of therapeutic massage and have identified specific points in the body where massage is most effective.

Massage for companion pets is currently a growing field. We all know everyday touch can bring our dogs comfort, but massage does much more than this: It triggers a response of the dog's nervous system, signaling the dog's body to heal itself. Massage focuses on the soft tissue of the body, including the muscles. It plays an important role in post-surgery and post-injury rehabilitation, as well as in the treatment of more chronic conditions, such as arthritis. Dogs with hip dysplasia, hygroma (a false bursa that occurs over boney areas and pressure points) arthritis, allergies, swollen joints and even dry, flaky skin can benefit from regular massage. Gingivitis (red inflamed gums) can also be treated with gentle, circular massage to the gums, which increases circulation.

When working with senior dogs, the therapist will perform a more thorough assessment of the dog's body than they might in younger animals at each massage to look for any changes, including any increased or decreased signs of tension or soreness. For some aging dogs, the massage sessions may need to be shorter and more frequent.

The massage can be performed on the floor with a soft dog bed or on a massage table. Most dogs prefer the floor; however, some like massage tables—tables are easier on the practitioner. It is important not to allow the dog to jump off the table on his own as injury can occur.

Overall body palpations should be done at each massage. The therapist will evaluate the dog for hot or cold areas, adhesions, tight fibrous bands of muscles and abnormalities, such as new lumps on the dog's body. An assessment should also include evaluation of the dog's gait and postural distortions.

Three different types of canine massage are commonly used on senior dogs:

Trigger-point massage utilizes a hands-on technique similar to that in acupressure. The massage begins like any other, with a scanning of the body for areas of tenderness that need healing. Once these points are located on the dog, the therapist will apply gentle pressure for 5 to 15 seconds and then lighter pressure to release the muscles and alleviate pain. This massage should be done by a trained massage therapist, one who is particularly adept in locating and releasing these trigger points. These are tender points on the dog and can be extremely sensitive if the area is pressed too firmly.

Therapeutic massage is relaxing, promotes general wellbeing, boosts the immune system and increases circulation and muscle tone. It can be performed for many medical issues. Unlike trigger point massage, which focuses on specific pressure points, therapeutic massage involves long strokes and kneading techniques used on the muscle layers, which causes toxins to be released from the tissues and supplies nutrients to the muscles. This is a great massage for making dogs more comfortable and creating a better overall quality of life for them.

Sports massage is utilized for the healthier, active senior dog. This massage is more intense than the others. A bit more pressure is used. A pre-sports massage is done before exercise. It is designed to prevent injuries by warming up the dog's muscles, which increases blood flow. The post-sports massage loosens the muscles and circulation after exercise, helping to prevent stiffness and soreness in the dog.

Massage isn't the only form of touch that can be beneficial to your senior dog. A therapist may also do some **stretching** with the dog, which assists with range of motion of the joints. As senior dogs slow down and do not stretch and contract the muscles in their bodies, the muscles shorten. If they remain in a shortened position, this often creates muscle and tendon weakness. A massage therapist will very slowly stretch the muscles in a deliberate fashion while the dog is relaxed. This must be done with very gentle movements; otherwise, injuries can occur. Passive stretches can be done with the dog lying or standing after the dog's muscles have been warmed up. A trained massage therapist can show you safe stretching techniques you can do with your dog at home to promote more range of motion and muscle health.

Acupressure is also an effective "touch" method. Acupressure is an extension of the ancient Chinese culture of acupuncture. They are both based on the same principles, utilizing the concept of energy flow within the dog's body. They seek to stimulate the points where energy meridians lie beneath the skin. Acupressure involves placing physical pressure on various pressure points of the body. In a gentle, noninvasive way, this pressure balances and releases the flow of blocked energy in the dog's body. It enhances circulation of blood and metabolic energies, improves the health of the lymphatic system, and boosts the dog's overall health and mental stability.

The benefits of acupressure include:

- Managing pain
- Strengthening the immune system

- Releasing cortisone, which alleviates inflammation and swelling
- Strengthening muscles, tendons and joints
- Releasing endorphins
- Increasing overall circulation
- Removing toxins
- Improving digestion
- Soothing dogs by reducing mental and physical stress

Acupressure can be used alone or in conjunction with other alternative remedies, such as massage. Dog owners won't have trouble finding a trained acupressurist, as they are widely available and usually are trained in canine massage or other alternative modalities. Traditional veterinary hospitals also often offer this and other complementary therapies at their facilities.

"Tui na" is another form of hands-on bodywork available for dogs, usually used in conjunction with acupressure. "Tui na" means "push and grasp." This is a form of Chinese manipulative therapy that resembles massage. It is very low risk and entails the practitioner kneading, rolling, pressing, gliding, cupping and rubbing areas between each of the dog's joints and acupressure points to open the body's defensive chi and get positive energy and blood moving in the muscles and throughout the body overall. Tui na is used to treat both acute and chronic musculoskeletal conditions in dogs, including joint, back and hip pain. It has similar benefits to massage and acupressure.

Craniosacral Therapy is another bodywork therapy founded by Dr. William Sutherland in 1935. The craniosacral system is basically comprised of the bones, vertebrae and sacrum around the skull and vertebrae. The connective tissue and fluid between them provide support and shock absorption to the brain and spinal cord. This connective tissue fluctuates along with the motion of the skull. Dr. Sutherland was struck by the idea that the cranial sutures of the bones where they meet were "beveled, like the gills of a fish." There is also a cycle and pulse, discovered by Dr. John Upledger, founder of the Upledger Institute. This pulse and other aspects of the system can be assessed by a trained practitioner through their hands.

There are many similarities in humans and dogs with the craniosacral mechanics. We both have 29 bones in the cranial system. These bones move in a rhythmical way with each other. The normal rhythm between the cranium and the sacrum is very crucial for the health of the dog and for the functioning of the musculoskeletal system. If there is dysfunction in this area from injury, stress or infection, it can create problems with the system and other neurological disorders.

Issues associated with cranial dysfunction are chronic ear and sinus infections, droopy eyes, excessive yawning, balance problems, head tilts and sometimes seizures.

Craniosacral therapy involves the therapist placing his or her hands on the skull or sacrum with a very light touch and allows them to tune into the craniosacral rhythm. The healer gently works with the spine and the skull and its cranial connective tissues. The restrictions of nerve passages are eased, spinal fluid is optimized and misaligned bones are restored to their proper position. The dog will become relaxed as the treatment progresses. Like other bodywork, it can help with the dog's immune, respiratory, lymphatic and nervous systems. The therapy can also be used for emotional healing and to improve general wellbeing.

Finally, **veterinary phytotherapy** is another hands-on treatment for musculoskeletal conditions. It combines movement analysis with manipulation of the musculoskeletal system. The therapist will first analyze the dog's gait, posture, and any range of movement abnormalities. The treatment involves the use of the therapist's hands on the dog's body and electrotherapy (electric muscle stimulation) to stretch the muscles and manipulate the joints. It is particularly beneficial for soft tissue injuries that involve the muscles and tendons.

After just one or two sessions of any of the hands-on treatments mentioned in this chapter, you should see immediate, positive results in your dog. Your pet should not feel worse after a treatment. Dogs have different needs than humans do, so it is important that the trained canine massage therapist be well versed in the anatomy and physiology of dogs before working on areas that have been stressed or injured. Without this knowledge, it is possible to make problems worse or even cause new injuries.

Make sure you hire a qualified, licensed or certified professional who has experience with your dog's issues, and always consult with your veterinarian before signing your dog up for any complementary therapy. Harm can come to your dog if done incorrectly. Below are a few resources with additional information and to assist you in finding a professional in your area.

Jennifer Kachnic has spent her life working and volunteering in animal welfare including fostering hundreds of dogs for local shelters through the years. She is a Certified Therapy Dog Handler for the American Humane Society, Certified Animal Reiki Practitioner and a Certified Canine Massage Therapist. She has been a regular contributor to a variety of pet magazines including Animal Wellness, Mile High Dog Magazine *and* Bark.

As President of The Grey Muzzle Organization, she leads volunteers around the country working to provide grants to animal shelters and rescues nationwide for senior dog programs.

SeniorDogBooks.com
PO Box 3331, Littleton, CO 80161
303-324-3911
Jenny@SeniorDogBooks.com

Facebook: Jennifer.Kachnic
Twitter: SeniorDogBooks
Blog: GreyMuzzle.org/Blog

My Favorite Resources:

Canine Massage – A Practical Guide by Hourdebaigt, Jean-Pierre
Balance Your Dog Canine Massage by Sue C. Furman, Ph.D
The Well Connected Dog – A Guide to Canine Acupressure
    by Zidonis, Nancy and Amy Snow
The Healthy Way to Stretch Your Dog by Sasha Foster and
    Ashley Foster, DPDT

American Holistic Veterinary Medicine Assn.
    www.AHVMA.org

Rocky Mountain School of Animal Acupressure and Massage
    www.RMSAAM.com

International Association of Animal Massage and Bodywork
    www.IAAMB.org

Acupressure Information
    www.Acupressure.com

Alternatives for Healing
    www.AlternativesForHealing.com

American Board of Veterinary Practitioners
    www.ABVP.com

The Association of Chartered Physiotherapists In Animal Therapy
    www.ACPAT.com

Upledger Institute
    www.UpLedger.com

Craniosacral therapy training
    Holistic Veterinary List
        www.HolisticVetlist.com
    Senior Dog Books
        www.SeniorDogBooks.com

11

Canine Chiropractic Care
with Andi Harper, DC, CAC

What is Chiropractic Care and is there a difference between Human and Animal Chiropractic Care?

How do I find a Certified Animal Chiropractor?

"Chiropractic is both treatment and prevention. It has much to offer, from improving the quality of life of the geriatric to enhancing the performance of the athlete and all patients in between ..."
– *The Canadian Veterinary Journal, October 1999*

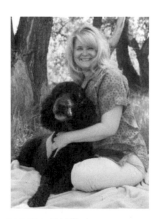

Chiropractic care focuses on diagnosing, treating and preventing nerve stress caused by distortions in the musculoskeletal system with special emphasis on the spine. This stress is known as a subluxation.

Subluxations can cause physical and emotional malfunction.

They are associated with loss of energy, pain, weakness, neurologic issues and disease of all types. This goes for any subluxation in any spine or body structure of the human, horse, dog or cat.

Chiropractic treatment emphasizes manual therapy, including spinal manipulation and other joint and soft tissue manipulation. The manual therapy can include either a hands-on method or the use of a hand-held, low-force mechanical adjusting device. Traditionally, it is assumed that a vertebral subluxation or spinal joint dysfunction can interfere with the body's function.

The origin of chiropractic is credited to D.D. Palmer during the mid-1890s. It was further developed by D.D. Palmer's son, B.J. Palmer, through research and clinical practice. Although the Palmers are known as the founders of current chiropractic care, adjustments have been used for thousands of years.

Chiropractic does not have a philosophy; it IS a philosophy, which encompasses the existence of universal intelligence that is an invisible force which brings organization to matter and maintains its existence. Chiropractic encourages and directs this innate intelligence to allow the body to heal itself. This was the original hypothesis that Hippocrates believed back in 460BC, which has remained strong to this day.

B.J. Palmer promoted the chiropractic profession and began adjusting animals back in the 1940s. Animal chiropractic is a broadening of human chiropractic with techniques developed to be able to treat animals. If you think animal chiropractic is something new, consider that in 1944 he wrote,

In the early days of chiropractic, we maintained a veterinarian hospital where we adjusted the vertebral subluxations of sick cows, horses, cats, dogs ...

The same philosophy, science and art are applied to the animal as to the human, with certain adaptations according to the variations in their anatomy.

Modern animal chiropractic for animals began in the State of New Jersey in the early 1980s when a group calling itself Options for Animals began working on dogs. The project was short-lived, as legal action was launched against one of the chiropractors by veterinarians in the state. The organization was later revived when veterinarian Dr. Sharon Willoughby enrolled and graduated from Palmer College of Chiropractic. Soon after that, "Options" opened a school for animal chiropractic.

Today, there are three schools in the United States, one in Canada and Europe. The courses are open to any qualified chiropractor or veterinarian. In most states/jurisdictions in the U.S. and Canada, completion of this program is mandatory for those who wish to practice animal chiropractic and become a certified animal chiropractor. Recognition of animal chiropractic as a separate professional entity began when the American Veterinary Chiropractic Association was established.

How Do I Know if My Senior Dog Needs an Adjustment?

The most common question I receive from pet owners is, "How do I know if my dog needs an adjustment?" The simplest answer is:

Whatever you would see your chiropractor for,
your pet should see their animal chiropractor for.

Specifically, for the senior group, it is time to see a chiropractor when they are having a hard time getting up from a seated or lying position, difficulty going up or down stairs, or trouble getting into or out of the car. They may be exhibiting generalized weakness or may seem "off" or just plain uncomfortable. Many owners report that their dog is fine one day and sore or lame the next. In most cases, owners report they have no idea what has occurred.

What Are the Benefits of Chiropractic Care for My Senior Dog?

There are numerous common stressful or traumatic situations that can cause abnormal or restricted movement to occur in the spine or a subluxation. When a subluxation occurs, the dog's spine loses its normal flexibility. This results in stiffness, which further leads to resistance and decreased performance. The most common symptom associated with restricted movement in the spine is pain, which can manifest itself in a variety of ways.

A surprising number of problems that may seem unrelated to a "back problem" actually are a direct result of a problem in the spine. All of the nerves that come out of the spinal cord exit between the individual vertebrae that make up the spine. When there is a vertebra that is not moving properly it puts pressure on the nerves that pass by it—which may result in problems seen further down the pathway of the affected nerve(s). These problems may be pain, spasm, lameness or weakness in another area of the body or even affecting an internal organ that is at the endpoint of the nerve.

According to the American Veterinary Chiropractic Association, chiropractic care is appropriate in the treatment of:

1. Neck, back, leg and tail pain
2. Muscle spasms
3. Disc problems
4. "Neurologic" or "Knuckling Over," most commonly seen in the rear leg(s)
5. Lick Granuloma, more common in the front leg(s)
6. Joint problems, limping/lameness
7. Injuries from slips, falls and accidents
8. "Sloppy Sitting," legs off to one side may be seen in your puppy or adult dog
9. Event or sports injuries
10. Post-surgical care, most commonly following TPLO (tibial plateau leveling osteotomy).
11. Bowel, bladder and internal medicine disorders
12. Maintenance of joint and spinal health

The above list goes for any dog, young or old, athletic or a couch potato, pure breed or mixed breed. Although listing old age as a disease process sounds unfair, a good portion of what is listed above is due to age and how the dog's body breaks down due to the aging process.

The Aches and Pains of Aging

Animal chiropractic practices consist of essentially two groups; one group is the dog athlete and the other is the senior dog. The majority of my practice is dedicated to making and keeping dogs comfortable through their golden years.

As dogs age, they move their weight forward to the front legs. No matter the size or breed, when they are young, they generally have about 60 percent of their weight up front and 40 percent in the rear. With age, they become more "front-loaded." This movement of weight to the front legs leads to many other symptoms including:

- pain and tightness between the shoulder blades;
- neck pain;
- weakness in the rear;
- tripping in either the front or the rear; and
- becoming what the vet world likes to refer to as "neurologic" in the rear, or knuckling and crossing of the back legs.

What does "neurologic" mean? Veterinarians love to throw this word around. As a pet owner, do you know what it means? I ask a lot of my clients that and they seem to have a vague idea, mostly that it is not a good thing. In the vet-world, it is not a good thing and most times, untreatable. In my chiro-world, it is exactly what I treat every day with wonderful results. What needs to be determined is what is causing the neurologic symptoms. The majority of the time it is a severe muscle spasm impinging on a nerve which then causes the signal to slow down.

The result is that we see knuckling of the paws, pain, weakness, tripping, and/or lameness.

Another side-effect of becoming front-loaded with age is cervical or neck pain. Half the time, a dog will present with neck pain as the primary issue. After two to four visits, the neck pain has resolved and the primary reason for it becomes apparent. When the lumbar spine or hips are painful, the body compensates with moving weight forward—the result is neck pain that flows through the dog. I tell owners all the time—you can almost cut off your dog's back leg and he will still want to go on a walk; but neck pain—it will affect them severely.

Most of the time, there is whimpering or crying out due to pain, this primarily occurs in the middle of the night because they are unable to get comfortable. Moving just the wrong way can cause a muscle to spasm resulting in a sharp stabbing pain. Ever wake up yourself after "sleeping wrong" and not being able to move your head? Can you recall the pain, a headache and/or feeling really bad associated with "sleeping wrong"? Now imagine the same for your dog. Moving just the wrong way can cause a muscle to spasm resulting in a sharp stabbing pain.

A lot of owners are very concerned about their dog and a trip to the ER vet is the next step. He is helpful in alleviating the pain, but little else is offered. X-rays, if taken, usually do not show a boney issue such as arthritis, but soft tissue *stuff*, like muscle spasm and inflammation, does not show up on x-rays. The ER vet usually recommends that they see their regular vet in the morning. This is where your certified animal chiropractor and chiropractic care comes to the rescue.

Chiropractic care is able to treat the entire neurologic system by stimulating joints and removing subluxations. In turn, the muscles are relaxed and pain and inflammation is relieved.

Can arthritis be treated with chiropractic care? Absolutely! Arthritis is the number one issue that chiropractors treat in humans and animals. What, exactly, is arthritis? Arthritis is inflammation of one or more joints—a joint is the area where two bones meet and involves the breakdown of cartilage. Cartilage normally protects a joint, allowing it to move smoothly. It also absorbs shock when pressure is placed on the joint, such as when your dog walks or runs.

Cartilage has very poor blood supply; it stays healthy with regular motion through the entire range of motion of the joint. Without the normal amount of cartilage, the bones rub together, resulting in arthritis. With arthritis comes pain, swelling (inflammation) and stiffness. Chiropractic adjustments return that complete motion of the joint to prevent arthritis.

For those senior dogs where arthritis is already present, chiropractic adjustment allows for more motion to be put into the joint, therefore reducing pain and inflammation. The boney changes cannot be reversed with adjustments—but the pain, stiffness and discomfort can be greatly reduced.

Many senior dogs are on medications to help with pain and inflammation. Not surprisingly, many medications can have adverse effects on dogs, including GI disturbance or liver issues. Chiropractic care works well in conjunction with medications. In many circumstances, it allows for the decreasing of drugs—a positive outcome for your dog's body. Of course, regular discussions and blood work with your primary veterinarian is advised before the reduction or elimination of prescribed medications.

Hip Dysplasia Affects Young and Old Alike

Does animal chiropractic help with hip dysplasia? Yes! Hip dysplasia in the simplest term is a form of arthritis that has developed over the dog's lifetime. Owners will often call wondering if their senior dog has developed hip dysplasia when they appear to be having trouble standing up from a sitting position, or sometimes it shows as reluctance to sit or sitting becomes very slow.

Canine Hip Dysplasia (CHD) is a condition which begins in young dogs, ages 9 - 18 months, with instability or a loose fit of the hip joint. The most common thing I hear from owners that makes me suspect CHD is their report that their one-year-old dog has a lot of trouble getting up from a lying position to a standing position or that they are "not big jumpers."

Hip dysplasia presents in young animals as instability of the hip joint. As the dog bears weight, the head of the femur (the "ball") comes out of the acetabulum (the "socket") as far as the joint capsule and ligament will allow. The joint capsule and ligament gradually get stretched, allowing the femoral head to come out of the acetabulum even further.

The result of the instability in the joint is abnormal wear and tear of the cartilage. Cartilage wear leads to the formation of bone spurs and joint capsule thickening, which are the characteristics of arthritis. The formation of arthritis is the body's attempt to help stabilize the hip joint and is visible on x-rays. Over the life of the dog, the arthritis progresses. However, radiographic signs of arthritis do not always correlate with how well the dog moves and their pain level. Presently, it is believed causes of hip dysplasia are usually hereditary. The incidence of hip dysplasia is greatest in large breed dogs.

The clinical signs of hip dysplasia are lameness, reluctance to rise or jump, shifting the weight to the forelimbs, loss of muscle mass on the rear limbs and pain when the hips are manipulated. Dogs may show clinical signs at any stage of development of the disease, although many dogs with hip dysplasia do not show overt clinical signs. A number of dogs experience pain at six to eight months of age but recover as they mature. As the arthritis progresses with age, some dogs may show clinical signs similar to people with arthritis including lameness after unaccustomed exercise or after prolonged confinement. If your dog is overweight, the problems will be worse.

You should seek veterinary advice on treating the pain and lameness with nonsteroidal anti-inflammatory drugs (NSAIDS). Concurrent treatment with a nutraceutical agent, chiropractic and/or acupuncture may also be recommended.

What Will My Dog's First Chiropractic Treatment Be Like?

Most animal chiropractors practice a manual technique with palpation of the spine and extremities. This palpation will reveal when a joint is not moving properly through a normal range of motion, if there is a subluxation, and if the dog is in need of an adjustment. Unlike people, dogs generally are not very good at staying in particular positions when being adjusted. Most certified animal chiropractors work with the dogs on the floor in any position that is comfortable for the dog. They will use their hands and adjust with a high-velocity, low-force thrust into the joint that is not moving properly.

Most dogs do very well with adjustments, although all bets are off if the dog is in a lot of pain. A muzzle may be needed to protect the dog, the owner and the doctor and may be needed until the dog is out of severe pain. Most dogs calm down once in a muzzle. Usually chiropractors will attempt to complete the treatment without a muzzle first.

Instead of using their hands, some certified animal chiropractors utilize an activator. This also tends to be the technique of choice for veterinarians that offer chiropractic adjustments. It is a small hand-held spring-loaded instrument which delivers a small impulse to the spine. The activator is categorized as an MFMA (mechanical force manual assisted) instrument which is generally regarded as a softer chiropractic treatment technique. It generates no more than 0.3 joules of kinetic energy in a 3-millisecond pulse. The aim is to produce enough force to move the vertebrae but not enough to cause injury.

Most commonly, the activator is used in combination with palpation of joints. The certified animal chiropractor or veterinarian will palpate the spine and other joints, locate the subluxation or joint that is not moving through the normal range of motion and instead of using their hands to adjust the joint, they will use the activator. This is a gentler adjustment, but the activator makes a clicking noise that some dogs do not appreciate.

The ArthroStim is new on the scene of animal chiropractic and is also a tool to make the adjustment more comfortable to the dog patient. The ArthroStim is an FDA approved instrument developed by IMPAC Technology in Oregon. It has been continuously refined and perfected over its 22-year history. It introduces energy/force/information to the body to realign segments and remove nerve pressure at a speed of 12 "taps" per second (12 hertz); it is a fast, accurate, low force and controlled adjustment.

In my practice, I offer a unique breakthrough approach to chiropractic care called Koren Specific Technique (KST). In late 2003, as a result of research and clinical experimentation, Tedd Koren, DC developed this improved form of chiropractic spinal care. When using KST in combination with the ArthroStim, your senior dog will receive gentle, specific correction of subluxation to the spine, structural and organ systems.

The benefits of Koren Specific Technique include:

1. Quickly and easily analyzes and adjusts the structural system of your dog for subluxations: cranial bones, TMJ, the entire spinal column, pelvis, pectoral girdle, sternum, coccyx, ribs, extremities—any time, anywhere.

2. Adjusts disks.

3. Immediately tells if the subluxation was corrected.

4. Is low force. Most patients actually like the adjustment instrument.

5. Gets results for the most difficult patients.

6. Is gentle enough to use on all ages—from puppies to seniors.

7. Allows the animal chiropractor to know exactly where to adjust (without x-rays, computers, MRI or other analytical equipment).

8. Tells immediately whether or not subluxation is corrected— NO MORE OVER-ADJUSTING (this is very important when your clients cannot talk to you).

9. Helps patients be more thoroughly analyzed than ever before, with the adjustments holding better and for longer periods of time.

How Will My Dog Be Feeling After Their First Adjustment?

How your dog will feel after their first adjustment runs the gamut, from "Wow, I feel great" to "Can we go home? I need to take a nap." Older dogs in general tend to be pretty tired after an adjustment and will often go home and go to sleep. They may even be sorer for 24 - 48 hours afterward. Some will even experience some loose stool (it should be no more than one bowel movement). All of this depends on what is going on and what medications are being prescribed by their veterinarian.

Chiropractic care is a holistic approach to many health and performance problems of dogs. Chiropractic does not replace traditional veterinary medicine and surgery but provides a complementary method of care.

How Do I Find A Certified Animal Chiropractor?

Animal chiropractic regulations vary considerably from state to state. Most states allow certified animal chiropractors to work on animals with a veterinarian present when the animal is adjusted. A few states allow a certified animal chiropractor to adjust an animal with a written referral. Others have absolutely no regulations at all. State regulations for what is considered a certified animal chiropractor and how an animal may be adjusted can be determined by contacting the chiropractic association for each state.

Most states that allow animal chiropractic require that veterinarians and chiropractors take a course that is certified by the American Veterinary Chiropractic Association (AVCA). It is an intensive 220-hour course taught in five modules with ongoing theoretical and practical examinations. The course outline includes anatomy, basic and advanced neurology, scientific validity, biomechanics, ethics and legalities, rehabilitation therapy, alternative and complementary therapy, modalities, basic chiropractic techniques for small animals and horses, case presentations, philosophy, alternative techniques, veterinary pathology, chiropractic pathology and advanced chiropractic techniques. There is also a sizable home study component.

Andi Harper, DC, CAC is a Doctor of Chiropractic and a Certified Animal Chiropractor. She completed five years of chiropractic-medical school in 2002 and immediately went on to do her post-graduate education in animal chiropractic. She completed the AVCA certified program in January 2003. Dr. Harper has also studied Reike and Craniosacral balancing - calming energy work that complements chiropractic care perfectly and works best on senior and geriatric patients. Dr. Harper specializes in the KST, which along with the ArthroStim™ tool introduces energy/force/information to the body to realign segments and remove nerve pressure. She adapted the technique for furry patients and is now getting phenomenal results. She is a graduate of National University of Health Sciences (2002) and holds her Certification in Animal Chiropractic from Options for Animals (2003), an AVCA-certified course. Dr. Harper travels to different veterinary and chiropractic clinics throughout the Denver-metro area.

Harper's Ridge Chiropractic Care, LLC.
www.HarpersRidge.com
303-518-3688
DrAndi@HarpersRidge.com
Facebook.com/HarpersRidge

My Favorite Resources:

American Veterinary Chiropractic Association
   www.AnimalChiropractic.org
Options for Animals
   www.AnimalChiro.com
Activator Methods
   www.Activator.com
ArthroStim
   www.ImpacInc.net
Koren Specific Technique
   www.TeddKorenSeminars.com
American College of Veterinary Surgeons
   www.ACVS.org
Information Center for Canine Arthritis
   www.Glucosamine-Arthritis.org
Email Group for People with Disabled Dogs
   www.AbleDogs.net

12

Traditional Veterinary Chinese Medicine with Erin Mayo, DVM, CVA

What is it and how can it help a senior dog?

Can Traditional Veterinary Chinese Medicine help with my dog's cancer?

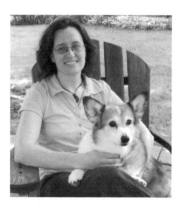

Traditional Chinese veterinary medicine (TCVM) is an ancient practice that has been gaining more popularity in the United States. Our geriatric pets can greatly benefit from these techniques, and even younger, healthy dogs can see improvements in energy, attitude, physical performance and overall quality of life using this practice.

TCVM does not address the animal as individual body parts as Western veterinary medicine does. Instead, a TCVM practitioner will look at the pet from a holistic viewpoint and treat accordingly.

In this respect, a TCVM practitioner can treat seemingly disparate conditions, such as a skin condition and vomiting, at the same time and sometimes with only one herbal formula. From the TCVM perspective, the body is seen as a whole, and symptoms of disease signal an imbalance within the dog, not just the one body system.

Let's Start from the Beginning—TCVM Basics

TCVM philosophy can be difficult to understand for the beginner. It is deeply rooted in Taoist teachings about nature and frequently uses metaphors to describe complicated metabolic processes in the body. Rather than trying to understand everything at once, it is best to start with the most basic concept of TCVM, that of *Yin* and *Yang*.

Yin and *Yang* represent the two extremes that are seen in the world and describe the nature of all things. *Yin* represents substance, cold, dark, sinking, moisture, night and femininity. *Yang* represents energy, warmth, light, rising, dryness, day and masculinity. These two forces exist in all things; one cannot exist without the other. Balance and harmony is achieved when *Yin and Yang* exist in equal amounts and intermingle.

The classic representation of these two forces is the *TaiJi* symbol.

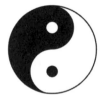

Yin is the black half, and *Yang* is the white half. This symbol shows how the *Yang* half is rising, and the *Yin* half is sinking. Both halves are equal in amount and are not separated by a straight line but a curved line, as if the halves are swirled. This represents how the two forces can mix together to create different combinations of light and dark, hard and soft and so on. The white dot and black dot represent how aspects of the opposite can be found in the other. It is the intermingling of the two forces that creates life.

These two forces naturally want to separate, much like the concept of entropy. The metabolic processes in the body, such as digestion and breathing, are all designed to bring these two forces together. When this occurs, *Qi*—otherwise known as energy or life—is created. Once created, *Qi* travels throughout the body to assist with metabolism and further mixing of *Yin* and *Yang*.

Bringing *Yin* and *Yang* together is an active process that requires constant effort on the body's part. Energy for this comes from oxygen in the air and nutrients in food.

> *When a body is in balance, it is able to utilize the energy from the air and food it takes in, combine this with* Qi *and bring together* Yin *and* Yang *to create more* Qi.

Qi then helps to power all the organs and important processes needed to extract energy from air and food. In this manner, a harmonious cycle is established.

Disruption of this cycle, anything that upsets the delicate balance of opposite forces, will result in signs of disease. From the Chinese perspective, treatment centers on re-establishing balance. Once balance is restored, the body can re-establish its natural harmonious cycle. A TCVM practitioner does not address individual signs of disease; signs of disease are used as guideposts to indicate the body's overall imbalance. In this way, Chinese practitioners do not heal disease. They help restore balance in the body, so the body may then heal itself.

The Aging Process and Disruption of Balance of *Yin* and *Yang*

As the body ages, the harmonious cycle of *Qi* production is often disrupted. This is most commonly the result of decreasing function of internal organs or declining amounts of vital substances, such as Essence. When *Yin* and *Yang* are not properly intermingled, less *Qi* is produced. The result of this process is inadequate *Qi* production; complete failure of the organs; and ultimately, death. Instead of a balanced cycle, a new cycle is established, one of slow decline. Imbalances can be expressed in a variety of ways, which accounts for the variety of disease symptoms. A TCVM practitioner will ask questions and examine the pet to determine what symptoms are present. The symptoms are then organized into a pattern of disease; this is known as pattern differentiation.

A commonly seen disease pattern in older dogs is "Kidney" deficiency. In Chinese medical theory, the "Kidney" is responsible for controlling urine. Unlike conventional medicine, Chinese medical theory also believes the "Kidney" is responsible for providing power and strength to the hind legs and controls the ears and the brain. As a dog ages and "Kidney" function decreases, the dog will often show symptoms of weak hind legs, confusion and decreased hearing. Conventional medical doctors would approach these as separate problems, but a Chinese medical practitioner would see them as a pattern of symptoms consistent with deficient "Kidney" function. In this manner, TCVM is able to address multiple disease symptoms by treating one imbalance.

Tools of the Trade – Acupuncture, Acupressure, Herbs and Diet

Acupuncture is the placement of fine needles at specific locations on the body known as acupoints. These acupoints are located along a series of channels that run throughout the entire body. Channels are conduits along which vital substances, such as "Blood" and *Qi*, travel. The stimulation provided by the needles can manipulate the flow of these vital substances.

> *Specific combinations of acupoints can relieve obstructions, draw* Qi *to an area of low concentration or drain it away from an area of high concentration.*

Acupoints can also have specific properties, such as influence over a specific body part or internal organ. Acupoint combinations, also known as point prescriptions, are tailored to the specific imbalance of each patient. It is possible that two patients with the same disease will receive very different point prescriptions because their overall imbalance of vital substances and organ function is different.

Now, if you are confused about *Yin, Yang* and *Qi*, let's look at acupuncture from a Western scientific perspective. Acupoints are located near bundles of nerve endings and capillaries (small blood vessels). When a needle is placed in the skin, the nerves and capillaries are stimulated. Locally, chemicals are released that increase blood flow to the area. Increased blood flow can help flush toxic substances out of the area or bring important cells to the area, such as those associated with the immune system. Stimulation of the nerve endings sends chemical signals to the spinal cord and brain. This can provide pain relief or even stimulate important metabolic functions in other locations of the body. It has been documented that stimulation of acupoints on the legs increases gastric acid secretion in the stomach. Clearly, the insertion of a tiny needle in the skin can have far reaching consequences throughout the entire body.

Acupuncture does not always need to be performed with a needle. Acupressure, for example, employs touch to stimulate acupoints. Lasers use light energy to stimulate acupoints. Other techniques can be combined with needles, such as electro-acupuncture. This technique utilizes electrodes that are attached to the needles, and low levels of electrical current are run between the needles. This method is frequently employed for more severe conditions, such as paralysis. Moxabustion is a technique that involves burning dried mugwort. The compressed herb can be held near the needle or attached to the needle and provides gentle warmth, or *Yang* energy.

Herbs work similarly to acupuncture. They can manipulate the flow of *Qi* and other vital substances in the body. They may also directly influence the function of specific organs or provide building blocks for the body to produce vital substances. From a scientific perspective, herbs and plant-derived medicinal products can produce powerful effects in the body.

Plants contain many chemicals, and the subtle interaction of these substances creates a wide variety of physiological effects. Ginseng, for example, has been shown to *increase* immune function in patients with poor immune function and *decrease* it in patients with overactive immune function. This is called "immunomodulation," otherwise known as the ability of a substance to adapt its physiologic effect to the situation.

This may seem like voodoo, but it is a documented ability of several different plant species. Scientists have yet to adequately explain this phenomenon; they speculate that the combination of the many chemicals, and other substances specific to the plants, may be responsible. This is why many herbalists argue that purifying specific compounds from plants for medicines is inappropriate; using the plant in its natural, whole state gives the best result.

Chinese herbs are almost never given individually; they are given in combinations known as formulas. There are thousands of formulas, some as old as Chinese medicine itself. The formula is designed to address a specific combination of symptoms and imbalances. Some formulas contain only three or four herbs, while others may have more than 20. Each herb is selected to address a symptom; or direct the other herbs to a particular location in the body; or even to decrease potential side effects.

In TCVM, diet, or food therapy, is another important treatment method. As the saying goes, "You are what you eat." Again, recommendations are always tailored to the specific patient and frequently center around temperature. All food has an inherent temperature: hot, cold and neutral. Relating this back to *Yin* and *Yang*, warm foods are more *Yang*, while cold foods are more *Yin*. If your dog is judged to be too hot (or *Yang*), cooling and neutral foods will be recommended, while hot foods are to be avoided. In this manner, food can be used to correct imbalances in the body, and if the imbalance is mild enough, food therapy is frequently all that is needed.

Examples of How TCVM can Treat Canine Geriatric Ailments

TCVM can be used to treat any disease, including those commonly seen in geriatric dogs, such as diabetes, kidney disease, skin conditions and cognitive dysfunction. Now that you have a general idea of what TCVM is and the variety of treatment methods a TCVM practitioner might employ, let's look at some examples of how this ancient medical practice may help our senior dogs. Two of the most common conditions seen in senior dogs are arthritis and cancer. TCVM may be used to treat both.

Arthritis

As our pets live longer, they are experiencing more troubles with degenerative joint disease, otherwise known as arthritis. Some dogs may have one painful joint, while others may feel pain in every joint. Over time, this pain may lead to disuse of the affected limb, loss of muscle mass or even loss of mobility. TCVM can be extremely helpful for this chronic and painful condition.

Acupuncture can provide pain relief without the side effects that may be associated with long-term use of anti-inflammatory medications. Needles may be placed near the painful joints as well as other locations on the body. Again, to the TCVM practitioner, painful joints can signify many different patterns of imbalance. This pain could be from stagnation of the flow of *Qi* in the joints, or it could be from the collection of pathological substances that will need to be broken down and flushed out of the body. These two patterns may stem from very different underlying causes, and it is the underlying imbalance that must be addressed.

> *If the underlying cause of the arthritis can be identified,*
> *it is possible to halt progression.*

Herbal formulas can also be prescribed to improve quality of life for dogs suffering with arthritis. Many of the formulas that are classically prescribed for arthritis pain contain plants with chemicals known to have anti-inflammatory effects. Just as with acupuncture, it is important to try to identify any underlying imbalance and address it. Herbs can be used as a single therapy, or in combination with acupuncture, prescription medications, massage and rehabilitation therapies. Some caution is warranted when combining herbs with medications, as there are documented interactions between some herbs and drugs. Make sure to always tell your TCVM practitioner about all your pet's medications before beginning a Chinese herbal formula.

Cancer

It is an unfortunate statistic that one in four dogs develops cancer in their lifetime. Older dogs have an increased risk. While some practitioners may claim to be able to cure cancer, this is not the result that most owners should expect.

> *Cancer should be considered something that can be treated as a*
> *chronic condition, like diabetes. It may not be possible to cure*
> *the condition, but it is possible to extend a dog's life while*
> *maintaining quality.*

TCVM can offer strategies to decrease pain, slow tumor growth, increase stamina, and even decrease side effects associated with conventional treatment. Either as a palliative, stand-alone treatment or in combination with other treatments, TCVM can offer hope even in the most hopeless situation.

Because cancer comes in all sizes, shapes and types, it is not possible to outline specific treatment protocols in this text. However, in general, acupuncture and herbal formulas can be useful for pain control and management of side effects from conventional treatments, such as vomiting and nausea from chemotherapy. Dogs that are suffering from lack of energy often feel revitalized after an acupuncture session. Many herbs have chemicals known to slow tumor cell growth. If the dog is receiving prescription medications, it is important to discuss them with your TCVM practitioner to ensure there will be no unsafe interactions between the herbs and drugs.

Acupuncture is very safe in almost any instance, but caution should be taken in cases of osteosarcoma (bone cancer). Some practitioners believe that acupuncture can worsen bone tumors. While there is no research evidence, some practitioners feel that acupuncture near this type of tumor can stimulate blood flow, and thus encourage faster growth of the tumor. Because of this, it is best to know exactly what type of cancer your pet has and where it is located before proceeding with acupuncture.

Food therapy is vitally important when discussing cancer treatment. Cachexia, or extreme weight loss associated with cancer, is a major problem when treating cancer in dogs. Feeding a dog a diet with adequate and appropriate calories will ensure that all the other therapies will have a better opportunity to work. Chinese food therapy focuses on feeding fresh whole foods. Raw is not necessarily the best in all cases. If you have a very "Cold" dog, it will have difficulty digesting a raw diet, because it is inherently cooling.

Dogs diagnosed with cancer benefit from a diet of lean meat, vegetables and fruit. Meat provides protein, vital building blocks to maintain lean muscle mass. Vegetables and fruit provide important vitamins and minerals, such as antioxidants, to aid the body in combating cancer.

Specific combinations of foods can be prescribed to address specific symptoms. In the case of the dog with "Cold" symptoms, that owner would be told to feed the animal warming proteins, such as chicken and venison; and avoid cool proteins, like turkey or fish. If an owner chooses to home cook for their pet, they should consult with their TCVM practitioner to make sure the diet meets the dog's nutritional needs as well as their treatment needs.

Conclusion

TCVM has much to offer a senior dog. This ancient medical practice uses methods that are safe, gentle, and most importantly treat the whole dog, not just the disease. Maintaining balance within the body ensures health and well-being. When this balance is lost, disease will occur. TCVM involves evaluating the entire dog, and treatment focuses on re-establishing balance so that the body can heal itself.

Dr. Erin Mayo graduated from the North Carolina State University College of Veterinary Medicine in 2002. She has worked in several general and emergency companion animal practices since graduation, but has always had a strong interest in holistic healing methods. She received her certification in veterinary acupuncture and Chinese herbal medicine from the International Veterinary Acupuncture Society. Currently, she owns a house-call based business providing holistic and integrative services for companion animals in central New Jersey. Her interests in veterinary medicine include traditional Chinese veterinary medicine, nutrition, geriatric medicine, hospice care, and integrative methods for treating chronic disease. Dr. Mayo's hobbies include reading, yoga and horseback riding. She shares her home with two coonhounds and three cats.

Veterinary Acupuncture and Alternative Therapies
VetAcupuncture@verizon.net
609-356-4611
www.VetAcup.com

My Favorite Resources:

Holistic Veterinarian List
www.HolisticVetList.com
American Holistic Veterinary Medical Association
www.AHVMA.org
The Chi Institute
www.TCVM.com
American Academy of Veterinary Acupuncture
www.AAVA.org

13

Energy Healing Therapies
with Jennifer Kachnic, CCMT, CRP

How can energy healing help my senior dog?

How can I get trained to do it?

Energy healing refers to the kind of therapy in which a person improves the flow of energy in an animal's body. It is the most natural form of healing available. While conventional medicine operates on the belief that treatments for diseases or ailments should be strictly biological, with energy medicine, the healer restores the patient's health by treating the mind, body and spirit. Studies are proving that treating all three elements provides the best results; thus, energy healing has gone from an

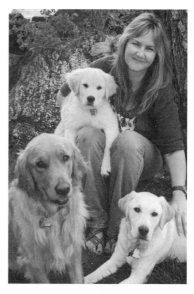

obscure curiosity to an integral part of leading-edge therapy in traditional medicine, and the idea that a universal energy field that encompasses us all exists is more accepted today than ever before.

Each life force is part of a vast energy field that extends beyond every being throughout the entire universe. This energy force is the mysterious glue that holds our universe together. It is through this energy that natural law is created and extends inward in all of us. During the process of going

145

through life and trauma, our energy flow can become disrupted; consequently, we can get separated from our core and soul, creating a state of imbalance in the body. The outcome can result in disease at a physical level.

Dogs are also spiritual beings—and subject to these same principles. If the flow of energy within a dog's body is disturbed, such as in times of stress, anxiety or tension, blockages can occur. These blockages can harm the body, mind or spirit and manifest into more serious illnesses. In energy healing, the healer acts as a conduit, directing energy into an ailing animal by visualizing and feeling the energy flow through his or her body into the dog. Certainly, there are skeptics out there who dismiss energy healing as a viable option, citing the placebo effect. Therapy with dogs, however, proves the placebo effect is not the explanation for the cures that result, as the dog is unaware of what is going on. Dogs just feel the positive intention of the healer.

Most energy healing is connected to the chakras (energy centers in the body). The main seven *chakras* are located along the spine, but there are many more present throughout the body. The healer, through calming his or her mind and body with controlled, slow breathing, can help to align and open up the chakras in the dog so they will be able to move in a balanced way, therefore allowing the energy to be distributed evenly throughout the dog's body.

Energy healing is noninvasive, nontoxic, economical and effective. It has measurable therapeutic value. It has been proven, for example, to help flush toxins from the body, release endorphins, relax muscles to increase circulation and also to elevate oxygen levels, which promote pain management. Healing energy therapies can be beneficial for dogs suffering from pain or disease, as well as stress. It is also very helpful in soothing dogs during the death and dying process. Energy healing also:

- Supports the body's natural ability to heal itself
- Vitalizes both body and soul

- Re-establishes spiritual equilibrium and mental wellbeing
- Balances the body's energies
- Adjusts itself according to the needs of the recipient
- Enhances senses
- Strengthens the vital organs
- Rejuvenates

The different techniques used in energy healing today are the result of the combined wisdom of therapies from various cultures around the world over the past centuries. There are many approaches; however, they basically all have the same effect. Here's a brief look at a few prominent techniques:

Qi-gong (pronounced chee-gong) is one of the oldest documented forms of energy healing. It is an aspect of traditional Chinese medicine, along with acupuncture and herbal medicine. The name comes from the combination of two Chinese words: *Qi*, meaning "life force energy" and *Gong*, meaning "the skill of working with cultivation."

This practice involves a combination of meditation, breath work and body movement, as well as visualization by the healer in order to guide the flow of *qi* into a dog's body. There are currently over 3,000 different types of Qi-gong practiced around the world—all can be divided into two categories.

Internal Qi-Gong builds the strength and optimizes the flow of energy within the healer's own body.

Medical Qi-Gong is external and applied by the healer to the patient, helping patients to heal themselves. It involves directing the energy into the dog's meridians and organs to release pathogens and bring the body into balance.

> *The role of the Qi-gong healer, as in all energy healing, is to open the channel in which energy is exchanged between the healer and the dog to assist in self-healing for the dog.*

Reiki (pronounced ray-key) is believed to have originated in Japan many centuries ago. The name consists of two Japanese words: *rei*, which can be translated as "the wisdom of God or the Higher Power," and *ki*, "the life force energy." Reiki practitioners undergo intensive training and receive "attunements" (blessings that are said to enhance the healing ability) that connect them to the Divine Universal Energy that then can be guided/channeled through their hands, breath, thoughts and eyes toward the client. Reiki is unique, as it uses special symbols and hand positions to invoke the flow of positive healing energy. The Reiki healer also gives attunements to the patient. The Reiki healer does not need to know what kind of ailment is being treated, as the energy flow is guided by its own innate wisdom.

Reiki energy gently and effectively opens blocked meridians and chakras and clears the energy in the body. Reiki helps the body/mind release stress and tension by creating deep relaxation, which in turn promotes healing and good health. The flow of these subtle energies can be felt as heat, coolness or calming sensations, as well as relaxation.

Master Reiki Teacher Sophia Paul says,
Most of my clients report a feeling of deep love and acceptance along with relaxation and stress reduction after a Reiki session. The skin will have a rosy glow, the breath will have slowed down and there is a luster to their eyes that they have not had previously. People are astonished at how nurturing and healing a Reiki session is. Reiki is noninvasive, gentle and suited for everyone, including dogs.

Healing Touch was developed by Janet Mentgen, a nurse who taught the first class back in 1989. She developed her technique using the philosophies and methods of many energy healers. Healing Touch is based on a heart-centered, caring relationship between the practitioner and the patient as they come together energetically to help facilitate healing. It is a biofield (magnetic field around the body) therapy and uses touch to influence a dog's body energy system to promote self-healing.

It works with the same energy systems as Reiki in a dog's body. This particular therapy is more structured than others. Because of the medical background of the founder, Healing Touch has been integrated into conventional medical and veterinary care as well as in nursing programs, medical schools and to a variety of other medical professionals.

Tellington Touch, also known as T-Touch, is the name for the energy healing technique developed by animal expert Linda Tellington-Jones in the late 1970s. Her methods include physical training exercises, body manipulation and light touching techniques. When performed, these procedures look like basic massage strokes, but unlike massage, T-Touch does not involve manipulating the animal's musculature. On the contrary, T-Touch is meant to stimulate the nervous system.

The therapist's stroke is very precise, with palm and thumb gently resting on the animal's body. The other hand is also placed on the animal's body to complete the flow of positive healing energy. Each specific stroke is designed to achieve different objectives, such as relaxation or relief of anxiety, and the therapy even facilitates positive behavior changes in the dog. I have seen dogs become much calmer for days after the treatment. T-Touch encompasses a number of skin lifting and touching techniques, as well.

As an energy healer and Canine Massage Therapist, when I treat dogs, it is not uncommon for me to experience strange feelings on my hands coming from the dog I'm working on. As I proceed, I can feel the energy around the dog's body allowing me to focus on the areas with the most resistance. Often, I find out after the treatment that a particular area of the dog's body from where I felt the most energy emanating had an injury or trauma previously. Usually, the caretakers are unaware the dog is still experiencing pain or discomfort in that area of his/her body.

The dog, in contrast to the healer, only feels energy flowing around its body. The sensation is so gentle, calming and relaxing, dogs usually fall asleep during the therapy.

After the treatment, dogs commonly feel more energized, less anxious, more confident and more connected to others.

I suggest offering water to the dog immediately after the treatment, as this is ideal in helping to facilitate the release of toxins from the dog's body.

Whatever energy healing technique is utilized, the processes are very similar. During energy healing, the healer stands or kneels next to the dog as the animal lies down. The healer's hands may or may not touch the dog during the treatment. The positive energy knows where it needs to go to bring balance and harmony to the dog's body and to help the body heal itself. It works in a nonphysical way through interconnectedness of body, mind and spirit. The dog receives the healing energy from the therapist, who visualizes healing for the dog with the understanding that what a person concentrates and focuses on creates reality.

With proper instruction and practice, anyone can perform energy healing on his or her dog to help facilitate healing and to improve the human-animal bond. We all have the capacity to tap into our own energy and help our dogs. Alternatively, dog caretakers can also seek treatments for their senior dogs from a trained practitioner or master.

Jennifer Kachnic has spent her life working and volunteering in animal welfare including fostering hundreds of dogs for local shelters through the years. She is a Certified Therapy Dog Handler for the American Humane Society, Certified Animal Reiki Practitioner and a Certified Canine Massage Therapist. She has been a regular contributor to a variety of pet magazines including Animal Wellness, Mile High Dog Magazine *and* Bark.

As President of The Grey Muzzle Organization, she leads volunteers around the country working to provide grants to animal shelters and rescues nationwide for senior dog programs.

SeniorDogBooks.com
PO Box 3331, Littleton, CO 80161
303-324-3911
Jenny@SeniorDogBooks.com

Facebook: Jennifer.Kachnic
Twitter: SeniorDogBooks
Blog: GreyMuzzle.org/Blog

My Favorite Resources

Animal Reiki Source
Training and practitioners
> *www.AnimalReikiSource.com*

International Association of Reiki Professionals
Reiki resources and practitioners
> *www.IARP.org*

National *Qi* Gong Association
Qi Gong resources and practitioners
> *www.NQA.org*

Qi Gong Institute Directory and general information
> *www.QigongInstitute.org*

Healing Touch for Animals
Training and practitioners
www.HealingTouchForAnimals.com

Healing Touch Program
Classes and practitioners
www.HealingTouch.net

Healing Touch International
Classes and practitioners
www.HealingTouchInternational.org

T-Touch Training and practitioners
www.CanineUnivesity.com
www.TTouch.com

Upledger Institute
Craniosacral therapy training
www.UpLedger.com

American Holistic Veterinary Medical Association
Natural healing for pets info.
www.AHVMA.org

Books

The Holistic Dog Book by Allegretti, Jan and Katy Sommers, DVM

Animal Reiki: Using Energy to Heal the Animal in Your Life by Fulton, Elizabeth and Kathleen Prasad

The Healing Touch for Dogs by Fox, Michael W.

Getting in Touch with your Dog – An Easy, Gentle way to Better Health and Behavior by Tellington-Jones, Linda

The Healing Promise of Q – Extraordinary Wellness through Qigong and Tai Chi by Jahnke, Roger

14

Working With Plants and Essential Oils with Frances FitzGerald Cleveland, EOS, HP

Can plants really help my senior dog?

What are herbs and how do I use them?

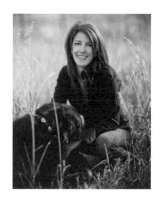

Although we would love to keep our young, energetic canine companions forever, it is inevitable that our dogs will get old. As they age, their systems will start to slow down, arthritis may set in and some older dogs may show signs of depression. You can help avoid or delay these conditions by starting your puppy out on a nutritious, healthful diet and maintaining it throughout his senior years. Then, when you notice he is beginning to show signs of aging, you can begin to incorporate plant medicine into his life, which can greatly enhance his quality of life.

The use of plants as medicine has been around for thousands of years. In written history, we find the study of plants dates back over 5,000 years to the Sumerians, who described medicinal uses for laurel, caraway and thyme. Ancient Egyptian medicine circa 1000 B. C. used garlic, opium, castor oil, coriander, mint and other plants. In India, Ayurvedic medicine utilized many herbs for medicinal effects, possibly as early as 1900 B. C.

In addition, there is evidence that the ancient Greeks and Romans used plants as medicine. During the Middle Ages, Hildegard of Bingen, a 12th century Benedictine nun, wrote a medical text about using plants called Causes and Cures. Although our modern mindset may at times lead us toward pharmaceutical options, the collected wisdom of our ancestors continues to be relevant. Today, we continue to study plants for medicinal use.

Animals have been instrumental in helping us discover some of this plant medicine. Many indigenous cultures studied animals, observing what plants they were eating. In the process, they discovered medicinal plants for human use. One example of this is Osha Root (Ligusticum porteri), also called bear medicine, a plant native to the western United States and Mexico. The story goes that Native Americans noticed bears rolling around in this plant, eating the roots and applying a root mash to injuries. They also observed bears seeking out this plant upon awakening from hibernation. The plant's respiratory and digestive cleansing properties may explain this; Osha Root is known for its powerful antiviral and antibacterial agents, used for bronchial infections and sore throats. (Because of osha root's popularity, it is now at risk of disappearing.) There are many other stories about indigenous cultures discovering their medicine by observing animals self-medicating with plants.

Today, wildlife biologists still find many new medicinal qualities in plants by observing animals in their natural habitats. We now call the process of animal self-medication zoopharmacognosy. Coined by Dr. Eloy Rodriguez, a biochemist and professor at Cornell University, the term refers to the process by which animals select and use plants, soils and insects to treat and prevent disease. The word zoopharmacognosy is derived from the roots "zoo" (animal), "pharma" (drug) and "gnosy" (knowing).

As this study continues, the use of plant medicine has developed into formal practices known as herbalism, medical herbalism, botanical medicine and aromatherapy (the term given for working with the essential oils from plants). In this chapter, I will draw on the combined knowledge from these disciplines to discuss the use of some herbs and essential oils that will benefit your senior dog.

Herb Basics and Uses

An herb is a plant that is valued for its flavor, scent and medicinal, spiritual or other qualities. The leaves, roots, flowers, seeds, resin, root bark, inner bark and berries are the most common parts of the plants considered herbs. The phytochemicals, chemical compounds that occur naturally in herbs, can have profound effects on the body.

An essential oil is a natural substance steam-distilled or cold-expressed from plants. The parts of the plant used for extraction are the flower, leaf, blossom, petal, resin, tree, bark, root, twig, seed, berries, rind and rhizome.

An essential oil is a complex mixture of over 100 organic chemical compounds. These chemical structures give the oil its smell, its therapeutic properties and, in some cases, its toxicity. Essential oils are 75 to 100 times more concentrated than dried herbs.

Some have referred to essential oils as the soul of the plant and consider them the plant's jewels.

Herbs and essential oils can be used as digestive aids, analgesics (relieves pain), anti-inflammatories (alleviates inflammation), antiseptics (prevents or combats infection locally), or bactericides (kills bacteria). Herbs and essential oils can also be bacteriostatic (inhibits growth of bacteria), cytophylactic (promotes cell rejuvenation when applied to the skin). They can promote circulation or act as a tonic for the system. These are just a few examples of the power of this plant medicine.

Providing plant medicine to our dogs as they age helps support their bodies, minds and spirits. This is also true of essential oils. During a dog's life, the hardest-working organs are the liver (it produces bile to help the digestion of fats and controls blood sugar levels), digestive organs and kidneys (they filter and eliminate waste from the blood).

> *There are many herbs and essential oils that can help support and nourish these systems in your dog's senior years.*

The primary herbs I first consider when working with senior dogs are dandelion root, devil's claw, gingko, hawthorne, licorice, marshmallow root, nettles, oatstraw, skullcap and yarrow. The primary essential oils I would initially consider are carrot seed, frankincense, ginger, grapefruit, helichrysum, rose, vetiver, violet leaf and yarrow. All of these have beneficial properties that can ease a dog's aging organs, and I would encourage you to investigate the particular effects of each oil or herb. At the end of this chapter, I've included brief descriptions of all these plants.

It's important to note that not all dogs respond in the same way to each herb and essential oil. With my two senior dogs, Merlin and Oscar, I noticed that their needs and desires for specific herbs and essential oils could be completely different at times. They each responded well to many of the primary plants listed above and others, but at different times during their senior years. Every dog is unique. By consulting professionals who have worked with animals in the field of herbalism and essential oils, you will find what your dog may need at that particular time.

When working with senior dogs, I design a plant formula based on their specific needs. While creating the formula, I consider the senior dog's overall constitution, its physical and emotional state, and what the veterinarian has told me about the dog. Medications or special diet are also important factors. Many Western and Chinese herbal formulas have proven effective and are prescribed for specific situations. Will your dog respond to one of these formulas? It is a high probability. Can the formula be designed more specifically for your dog? Yes, I believe it can.

When I was designing herbal and essential oil formulas for my senior dogs, they showed me that their needs changed from time to time. As a particular condition would flare up, I would adjust their formula. For example, when their tendinitis would flare up, I would focus on plants that would help to increase circulation and move stagnant blood. I also worked with essential oils that would complement this process, such as violet leaf, carrot seed and yarrow.

Merlin, a Black Labrador and Great Dane Mix...

In addition to using plant medicine for my senior dogs, I also incorporated other healing modalities to complement the work I was doing. For example, when we adopted Merlin, he was a year old. Merlin was badly abused as a young puppy and was rescued from this environment at the young age of six months. His body had taken a substantial amount of abuse. He had a broken left hip and broken right shoulder. Merlin's shoulder healed, but his hip was not healing very well, so the veterinarian hospital opted to do a Femoral Head and Neck Ostectomy. This operation consisted of taking off the head and neck of the femur. In Merlin's case, it was done to eliminate the head and neck of the femur bone from rubbing the fracture in his hip.

I knew that as Merlin approached his senior years, his very large body would have trouble. When he was eleven, his body started to fall apart, and the herbals I had formulated for him were no longer helping with the pain. His right hind leg, the "good leg," was starting to give out. Our veterinarian prescribed aquatherapy and an orthopedic brace to support his right leg. We also switched him to conventional pain medicines Tramadol, Gabapentin and Deremaxx. To counter the potential side effects of these conventional drugs, I formulated an overall body support herbal blend for Merlin. This blend supported his liver, kidneys, heart, nervous system and digestive system. For an entire year Merlin, went to his aquatherapy every week, which consisted of 30 minutes on an underwater treadmill, received massages every two weeks and wore his brace to go on long walks. His quality of life was greatly improved with all of these therapies.

Merlin passed away suddenly at the age of 12 from septic shock, but his body, mind and spirit were strong. At the end of this chapter I have included the herbal formula we worked with during Merlin's last year of life.

Drawing upon the practice of zoopharmacognosy and the ancient traditions of plant medicine, we can keep our dogs healthy and happy throughout their lives and, especially, in their senior years. The plants are here to help us and our dogs maintain a vibrant quality of life.

> Remember the Magic Formula:
> Healthy Diet + Exercise + Plant Medicine + Love =
> Healthy Happy Old Dog

Brief Definition of Primary Herbs:

Dandelion Root (Taraxacum officinale): One of the best liver and blood cleansing herbs. Dandelion root helps with hepatitis, jaundice, cirrhosis, as well as skin conditions, such as rashes, eczema and other skin eruptions (especially when combined with burdock seeds and calendula). It acts on the digestive system by stimulating the secretion of bile, which assists in digestion and elimination. It dissolves gallbladder and kidney stones and regulates blood sugar in diabetes and hypoglycemia. Dandelion root also gently promotes lymphatic activity.

Devil's Claw (Harpagophytum procumbens): Soothes pain and is a great anti-inflammatory. Very effective on arthritis in combination with glucosamine, chondroitin sulfate, cat's claw, yucca root and boswellia.

Gingko (Ginkgo biloba): Improves blood circulation and helps with vascular deficiency, which often occurs in old age. Many studies have shown that gingko helps to improve blood circulation in small blood vessels, and many of these types of vessels are found in the brain, ears and extremities.

Hawthorne (Crataegus spp.): A proven tonic to the heart and vascular system. Helps to stimulate circulation and move stagnant blood.

Licorice (Taraxacum officinale): A soothing herb. Helps with inflammatory conditions of the digestive system, such as canker sores, gastritis, peptic ulceration and excessive acid problems. Licorice's demulcent and healing properties also help with arthritis, inflamed joints and some skin problem. Licorice root should be used in moderation and for short periods of time. Excessive consumption of licorice is known to be toxic to the liver and cardiovascular system and may produce hypertension and edema.

Marshmallow Root (Althea officinalis): Useful whenever a soothing effect is needed, as marshmallow root protects and soothes the mucous membranes. It's a wonderful anti-inflammatory herb, particularly for infections or inflammation of the mouth, throat, kidneys, intestines, urinary bladder or urethra. An exceptional demulcent that lubricates the body, protecting against irritation and dryness, it settles acid indigestion, soothes dry cough, colitis and ulcers, lung inflammation, sore and irritated joints and the urinary system.

Nettles (Urtica dioica): Nettles' key use is as a cleansing and detoxifying herb. It has diuretic action, possibly due to flavonoids and high potassium content, and increases urine production and the elimination of waste products. Nettle's high mineral content helps support the kidneys.

Oatstraw (Avena sativa): Excellent nervous system tonic. Helps to improve and regulate nerve transmission. When fed in small amounts, it has a calming effect on chronic nervousness, and when given to debilitated animals, it tends to stimulate the nervous system. A wonderful tonic for aging dogs.

Skullcap (Scutellaria lateriflora): Skullcap is taken mainly as nervine tonic and for its restorative properties. It helps nourish the nervous system and calms and relieves stress and anxiety. Its antispasmodic action helps conditions where stress and worry cause muscular tension. As it relaxes nervous tension, it renews and revives the central nervous system. It may be used for all exhausted and depressed conditions.

Yarrow (Achillea millefolium): Infamous for its wound-healing abilities. Also an effective vasodilator and vascular tonic. Its flavonoid content helps to dispel small blood clots and as a result increases circulation. Yarrow also has anti-inflammatory and analgesic properties and is a nice herb for the respiratory, urinary and digestive tracts, as well as for the liver and skin.

Brief Definition of Primary Essential Oils:

Carrot Seed (Daucus carota): This oil has a cleansing effect on the mind and may help to relieve feelings of stress and exhaustion. It is considered an excellent blood purifier, due to its detoxifying effect on the liver. Carrot Seed is known to increase red blood corpuscle, so it has traditionally been used to boost the general action of all organs.

Frankincense (Boswellia carteri): Excellent effect on the respiratory system. Eases shortness of breath and is useful to asthma suffers. Helps to clear the lungs. Very calming and revitalizing for the nervous system, making it helpful for nervous tension and exhaustion. May be useful as an anti-depressive.

Ginger (Zingiber officinale): This oil is warming to the emotions. It sharpens the senses, aids memory and stimulates circulation. It is very cheering and is indicated for tiredness. Ginger's analgesic properties relieve arthritic pain, cramps, sprains and muscle spasms. Stimulating yet grounding, ginger also tones and settles the digestive system, promoting secretion of gastric juices. It helps with nausea, travel sickness and rheumatic pain.

Grapefruit (Citrus x paradise): A mild diuretic and stimulant to the spleen and lymph, this oil helps the body eliminate excess fluids and break down fats. It can relieve abdominal distention, constipation and nausea. On a psychological level, grapefruit eases feelings of tension, frustration, irritability and moodiness.

Helichrysum (Helichrysum angustifolium): Facilitates healing with its anti-inflammatory and antiseptic, cytophylactic properties and is effective for cuts, burns and wounds. Helps to rebuild tissues and energizes the organs, improving the general flow of the meridians. Aids in regulating blood pressure. Helps with aches and pains and with rheumatism. Other properties include expectorant (facilitates removal of mucus from the respiratory system), fungicidal (combats fungal infection), hepatic (tones and aids the liver's functions) and nervine (provides strengthening and toning to the nerves and nervous system).

Rose Otto (Rosa centifolia): A great anti-depressant that helps with nervous tension, trauma, fear and anxiety. It also eases anger, resentment, sadness, grief, or disappointment and other forms of stress. Rose otto is very useful for dealing with behavioral problems and has a tonic action on the heart by activating sluggish blood circulation as it helps to tone the capillaries. Balances and strengthens an emotionally upset stomach. Helps to clear the liver of toxins.

Violet Leaf (Viola odorata): Known to strengthen and comfort the heart. Contains salicylic acid, a natural painkiller. Helps with nervous exhaustion. This oil will not dull the senses; rather, it will help keep the animal in control, maintaining inner strength that would otherwise be depleted. Helps with poor circulation, rheumatism.

Vetiver (Vetiveria zizanoides): Seems to settle the nerves, helping to soothe states of irritability, anger and hysteria and instilling a more centered feeling. Vetiver revitalizes the body by fortifying the red blood corpuscles, which are crucial in transporting oxygen to all parts of the system. Increased blood flow can alleviate muscular aches and pains, and vetiver is said to be useful in cases of rheumatism and arthritis. Also helpful in cases of insomnia.

Yarrow (Achillea millefolium): Helps with hypertension, insomnia and stress-related conditions. Yarrow tones the skin and aids the healing of acne, burns, cuts, inflammations, rashes, wounds and scars. Balances the nervous component of digestion; improves absorption and digestive secretions, and helps with colic and flatulence. Stimulates bile; aids in digestion of fats, and encourages appetite. A great analgesic and anti-inflammatory. Yarrow is a beautiful oil which heals wounds on both physical and emotional levels. I have found many abused animals are very attracted to this oil.

Merlin's herbal formula for overall body support while on conventional pain medication included:

Primary herbs:
Plantain
Milk Thistle
Nettles
Dandelion Root

Secondary herbs:
Hawthorne
Cat's Claw
Oatstraw
Astragalus

Supporting herbs:
Yarrow
Ashwaganda
Celery Seed
Licorice

Essential oils Merlin would choose from:
Carrot Seed
Grapefruit
Rose
Violet Leaf (he chose this oil every time it was offered to him)
Yarrow

Oscar, a 12-year-old Black Labrador and Golden Retriever Mix, was diagnosed with arthritis in both front elbows and tendinitis in both front shoulders. In addition to the herbs and essential oils, Oscar is on Adequan, has massages every two to three weeks and receives laser treatments when he has a bad flare-up.

Oscar's Current Herbal Formula includes:
Primary Herbs:
Hawthorne
Gingko
Cat's Claw
Devil's Claw
Dang Gui
Safflower

Secondary Herbs:
Rose Hips
Dandelion Root
Oatstraw
Skullcap
Nettles

Supporting Herbs:
Yarrow
Tumeric
Licorice
Red Clover
Spirulina

Essential oils Oscar chooses from:
Carrot Seed
German Chamomile
Grapefruit
Helichrysum
Rose
Violet Leaf (he chose this oil every time it was offered to him)
Yarrow

Please note that this is only general information. **Too much of any type of medication can be toxic**. Please carefully study the plants you plan to use to support your senior dog and consult your veterinarian. Make sure the plants you choose work with the diagnosis, treatment plan and prescriptions your veterinarian is providing to your senior dog.

> NOTE: The lists addressing some of the properties of essential oils and herbs have not been evaluated by the FDA and, as such, shall not be construed as medical advice implied or otherwise. No claims are made with respect to treatment of any diseased condition and no attempt is ever made to dissuade individuals from seeking medical treatment for any condition. In addition, this equipment, technology and products have not been evaluated by the FDA, nor are they intended to treat, cure, mitigate, diagnose or prevent any illness or disease.

Frances Fitzgerald Cleveland has extensive experience in the realms of health and behavior as it relates to both animals and humans. She obtained certification from the Institute of Dynamic Aromatherapy and the International School of Animal Aromatics. Frances studied in England with Caroline Ingraham, the pioneer of Animal Aromatics. Frances is an apprentice of Rosemary Gladstar, world renowned author, herbalist and teacher, and has completed the intensive Apprenticeship Program and the Science and Art of Herbalism Program in the didactic, therapeutic, laboratory and fieldwork in herbalism. She is also a graduate from the University of Connecticut receiving a BA in Journalism and Environmental Science.

Frances recently trained zookeepers in the use of essential oils on animals. Her groundbreaking Animal Aromatherapy work at The Denver Zoo with the Orangutans, Gorillas and Black Crested Macaques was covered in the Denver Post and L.A. Times. Frances' work has also been written about by the Rocky Mountain News, Associated Press, The German Press and a featured guest on Animal Radio.

FrogWorks, Inc.
Natural Healing with Plants and Essential Oils for You
and Your Animals
Littleton, Colorado
877-973-8848
www.ffrogworks.com
frogworks@att.net

My Favorite Resources:

The Way of Herbs by Tierra, Michael

The Encyclopedia of Essential Oils by Lawless, Julia

The Complete Herbal Handbook for the Dog and Cat
by de Bairacli Levy, Juliette

Herbs for Pets by Tilford, Gregory L and Wuff Mary L

Veterinary Botanical Medicine Association
www.AAVA.org

15

Laser Therapy
with Brian A. Pryor, Ph.D.

Can laser therapy help with my dog's arthritis?

What does a treatment cost?

"You are going to LASER my dog?" Yes.

Today, lasers are being used by many veterinarians in the treatment of your four-legged companion. We are accustomed to hearing of lasers being used in applications as diverse as telecommunications to manufacturing computer circuit boards. Lasers are used to treat pain and inflammation in world class athletes, race horses and yes, household pets. They have been used for

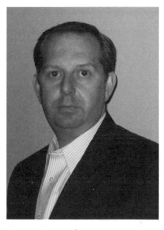

advanced medical applications for over 35 years. Ever since their invention, lasers have been a cool device in search of an application.

Medicine is one of many areas where lasers have made a considerable impact: vision correction, general surgery, lithotripsy, hair removal, cataract removal, wrinkle reduction and tattoo removal are just a few of the common uses for lasers today. Professional sports teams are regularly utilizing this technology on elite athletes in order to keep them healthy and in the game.

A relatively new application is the use of lasers for the relief of pain, the reduction of swelling and the healing of wounds. This is a unique use of laser light, due to the noninvasive nature of the treatment. Many laser applications use the intense energy which a laser can deliver to ablate or cut biological tissue. Therapeutic lasers, in contrast, work without any damage to tissue; the treatments are painless and quite enjoyable. Simply pass the laser over the body part and the pain goes away and the healing starts. Almost sounds too good to be true. Laser therapy is now being used by top doctors around the world.

The concept of laser therapy has been around for many years. It was first demonstrated during an unrelated animal study. Researchers noticed that mice exposed to the laser grew hair at a faster rate than the untreated mice. This led to the investigation of relatively low energy lasers on biological tissue. There have been thousands of studies documenting the effect laser light has on different types of cells, tissue and conditions. Until recently, the full potential of this exciting application hasn't been fully realized due to the expense of lasers, their size and the available power. Advances in technology and manufacturing now allows for suitable systems to be available for clinicians to use in their offices, or even portable enough to use in the field. There are now lasers being used to treat deep muscular\skeletal conditions on people, dogs, cats—even elephants. These treatments are quick, effective and of relatively low cost.

Today's veterinarian has access to this advanced laser technology, which can make a big difference in the care of older canines. Aging dogs are prone to arthritis, stiffness and other painful conditions just like we are as we age. Pain medications and anti-inflammatory drugs can have some very serious side effects on dogs, and long-term use of these medications is not ideal. Laser therapy is a safe, drug-free alternative to treat many common conditions, including arthritis.

Older dogs can display pain in different ways and often compensate for the pain by favoring one side while walking. Pet owners will often note reluctance by their pet to climb stairs or hesitancy to jump in the car. These symptoms need to be addressed as soon as possible, as this behavior can lead to increasing problems.

When started early, laser therapy treatments will start the healing process, reducing possible long-term problems, which may require the use of pain medications or even a major surgery like a joint replacement. Treating conditions early is the key. Pain can limit physical activity, which affects behavior, weight and general well-being. Weight gain will exacerbate any joint problem much faster.

By relieving the pain, your dog will remain active, alert and stay a healthy and happy member of your family. Lasers are now playing a greater role in providing this relief.

How Does It Work?

Although the treatments themselves are quick and easy, it isn't quite that simple if you look at the complex biochemistry which is taking place at the cellular level. The type of laser being used for laser therapy has the optimal wavelength, or color, to penetrate skin and get therapeutic light deep into the body.

As a child you probably put a flashlight up to your hand or even in your mouth. What happened? You saw a red glow through your cheeks. The green and blue components of the white light are absorbed by your tissue, and only the red light goes right through our tissue. Longer wavelengths in the near infrared go even deeper. Certain red and infrared wavelengths of light can also enter cells in our body and affect their behavior in a positive way. This is called photobiomodulation since we are using 'photons', the smallest unit of light, to 'modulate' cellular activity.

These photons are absorbed by chemicals in the mitochondria of the cells. This light energy then inspires production of adenosine triphosphate (ATP) in the cell. ATP is the fuel, or energy, our cells need for repair and rejuvenation. Impaired or injured cells do not make this fuel at the optimal rate. The laser interaction increases ATP production leading to healthier cells, healthier tissue and healthier animals.

Of course, there are many different types of cells in the body: muscle cells, nerve cells, skin cells, etc. Research is continually being performed on the laser's benefit to each particular type of cell. For example, laser therapy has recently been shown to have positive effects on nerve cells. Laser 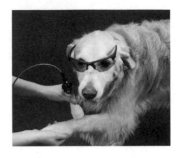 therapy changes the conduction of nerve cells which is one way the laser reduces pain and also aids in the actual repair of damaged nerves. This exciting field is continuing to grow, adding to the number of applications that address and improve many common health conditions. Your veterinarian will utilize protocols developed to treat the particular type of condition specific to your dog and the depth of the affected tissue.

Therapeutic lasers are being used for many conditions seen every day by your veterinarian. The following are the most common conditions in which the laser can help the older dog:

Joint Pain/Arthritis

It is often hard to locate the exact source of musculoskeletal pain in older canines. The pain can be associated with impairment of several joints or even the entire back. In these cases, laser therapy is a great treatment option since multiple areas can be treated in a short period of time. If your dog is having problems walking or getting up from a lying position, he may have hip problems. It is not uncommon that he will also be experiencing pain in the legs and the back.

The therapeutic laser can be applied to all affected areas in order to increase blood flow and reduce the pain as well as the inflammation. As a result, the surrounding muscle will be less stiff, pain will be reduced and the dog's range of motion improved.

As dogs get older, arthritis is more and more prevalent. Especially in the larger breeds, although any dog of any age can experience painful joints. Osteoarthritis causes severe inflammation in joints, leading to restricted movement and extreme pain. Laser therapy can play an important role in the management of osteoarthritis. Your veterinarian will use the laser to reduce swelling, allowing your dog to move better and with reduced pain. This improved movement will allow for additional exercise which, in turn, will enable joints to move and help keep the symptoms at bay. When managing osteoarthritis, it is important to take a comprehensive treatment approach which will include laser therapy, exercise, weight control, supplements and possibly medication.

Post-Surgical Incisions and Wound Healing

In the case of post-surgical pain reduction and wound healing, the laser is used over the surgery site. This is a very short treatment, typically less than two minutes. These treatments can improve the comfort of your dog after surgery. Post-surgical pain leads to discomfort which can be a major reason for an animal's delayed recovery. As soon as immediately after surgery, the therapeutic laser can be used in order to help with discomfort and to jump-start the healing process. Your dog will be much happier and have more range of motion. This laser treatment can reduce the need for pain medications. You will notice that the surgical incision will heal quickly; there will be less irritation to the area and very little scarring. As a result, your dog will experience less biting, licking and scratching of the area which will reduce the possibility of infection and/or re-injury at the surgical site.

A similar application to treating a surgical site is the treatment of a wound, whether it is acute trauma or a chronic wound such as a Lick Granuloma. In acute applications, the bleeding will be stopped and the wound will be cleaned; then the entire wound and the surrounding tissue will be treated with a short laser treatment. This treatment will lessen the discomfort caused by the trauma as well as stimulate the healing response leading to rapid and complete resolution of the wound.

Physical Therapy and Rehabilitation

Laser therapy has become an integral part in the rehabilitation of pets. Rehabilitation and physical therapy is now a standard in veterinary medicine, much like it is in human medicine. Getting the body moving after surgery or injury is often critical for optimal healing. Laser therapy will be used to make this motion less painful and easier. It will reduce the swelling and increase blood flow to the repaired tissue, shortening healing times. Rehabilitation of many conditions will include laser therapy and also incorporate many other important components such as water treadmill, exercise ball, electric stimulation, bracing, etc. Compliance is the key for a successful recovery.

What Will Happen When Your Dog Gets Treated?

Treatments are often performed by the veterinary technician. Treatments may be done on an examination table or as the dog is comfortably lying on the floor. Some practices even have a spa-like environment where your dog will lie on a sofa or plush bed. The treatment times will vary based on the size of the dog and the condition being treated. Typical treatments will take five to ten minutes for an average-size dog. For a more superficial condition such as a post-surgical incision or a wound, the treatment times will be very short, one or two minutes. For a deeper condition like hip dysplasia or an arthritic condition, longer treatment times are needed. The weight and the body condition will also determine how long a treatment will take. Since the laser will need to penetrate more tissue on a larger dog, the laser will either need to be used at a higher power or a longer treatment time.

There is no need for sedation or clipping of the dog's fur.

> *The treatment is very soothing and most animals will relax*
> *once the treatment is started.*

It is common for dogs to fall asleep during therapy. Some treatments will be done with the laser probe in contact with the skin. This will allow for excellent light penetration as well as a comforting or massage-like sensation for the dog. These treatments are also available for you, if you are feeling a little jealous (see your doctor). Your dog will feel a soothing warmth as part of the treatment. Eye protection will be worn by the laser operator and anyone in close proximity to the laser probe. The eyes of the animal will be directed away from the treatment area or covered with a towel or eyewear. The clinician will move the probe over the area of treatment to assure the laser is being delivered to the area which needs improvement. It is common that multiple joints will be treated during one laser treatment session.

What Can You Expect After Your Dog Has Been Treated?

You may notice your dog a little more comfortable after just one session with considerable differences being seen after about three treatments. Typically, laser therapy will be scheduled every other day for the initial treatments of more chronic conditions. Most conditions will need, on average, six total treatments to get a healing response. For chronic conditions, eight to twelve treatments may be needed, with the possibility of ongoing maintenance treatments on a monthly basis. Chronic conditions which have persisted for a long period of time can be challenging to treat, but hang in there. If progress is being seen, stick with the treatment recommended by your veterinarian as this new technology can make a significant difference in the health of your dog.

As discussed previously, the earlier treatment can be started, the better the outcome. Once conditions become chronic, results will take longer and medication may be needed in conjunction with the laser therapy.

How Much Will It Cost?

The costs of laser therapy sessions are based on the type of condition being treated. For a post-surgical treatment the price may be added into the overall cost of the surgery, or as an additional charge of $10 to $40. Longer treatments for an arthritic case will cost more, and depend on the length of treatment time. The average price per session is around $55. Many practices will offer laser therapy packages which may include multiple sessions for one fee.

If your dog is experiencing pain or discomfort, you should consult your veterinarian as soon as possible. Once your pet is diagnosed, laser therapy is a great treatment option due to the ease of treatment and the lack of side effects. The use of this proven technology can reduce or even eliminate the need for potentially harmful medications. Therapeutic laser treatments can help manage the joint pain that sets in as your dog gets older, keeping your companion moving, which is an important part of healthy aging. You should ask your veterinarian if therapeutic laser treatments can be beneficial for your furry friend.

Brian A. Pryor, Ph.D. is a founder and the Chief Executive Officer of LiteCure, LLC in Newark, DE. He completed his undergraduate studies in Mathematics and Chemistry at Salve Regina University in Newport, RI. He then continued his studies at the University of Pennsylvania where he received a PhD in Physical Chemistry. His thesis work was developing lasers and laser spectroscopic techniques to study molecular structures and interactions. He has published over 30 papers in the areas of chemistry, physics, laser development and their usages including laser applications in medicine. In addition to medical laser development, he has aided in the development of various laser sources for applications in semiconductor manufacturing, telecommunications and military operations. Over the past 10 years, he has studied how light and lasers interact with tissue, leading to the development of medical devices in the areas of aesthetics, diagnostics, and therapy.

Dr. Pryor has been the principle investigator in many research studies and developments sponsored by National Institutes of Health, US Department of Defense, and the National Institute of Standards and Technology. He has recently published a book entitled Clinical Overview and Applications of Class IV Therapy Lasers *and a recent book chapter entitled "Advances in Laser Therapy for the Treatment of Work Related Injuries" in the book Current Perspectives in Clinical Treatment and Management in Workers Compensation Cases. Dr. Pryor frequently lectures about light uses in medical applications.*

Brian A. Pryor, PhD. President and CEO of LiteCure
1-877-627-3858
www.Litecure.com
BrianP@Litecure.com

My Favorite Resources:

Email Group for People with Disabled Dogs
www.AbleDogs.net

Senior Dog News & Resources
www.SRDogs.com
www.DogWise.com

Dog Blogs
www.BlogPaws.com
www.BlogPark.com
www.SeniorDogBooks.com/Blog
www.AllThingsDogsBlog.com

16

Homeopathy Basics
with Marcie Fallek, DVM, CVA

Can homeopathy help with my dog's chronic illness?

Can it also help with emotional problems?

Homeopathy has its roots in ancient Greece, but was rediscovered by an 18th century German physician, Dr. Samuel Hahnemann.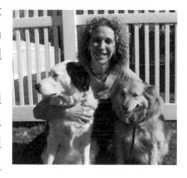

Disillusioned with the conventional medicine of the day, Hahnemann sought a better means of alleviating suffering and restoring the health of his patients. It is a true holistic medicine, in the sense that it treats the individual mentally, emotionally and physically. This is the antithesis of conventional medicine, which aims merely to suppress the physical manifestations of disease, as if it were an entity in itself, independent from the person or animal.

Homeopathy understands the truth that the 'dis-eased' state is a reflection of the inner imbalance of the individual, and that when you have restored that imbalance or disharmony, the physical symptoms will simply melt away. It treats the whole individual, not only the various diseased parts. A homeopath understands that symptoms are there for a reason, and merely removing them not only doesn't cure, but ultimately weakens and damages the individual, as it does with dogs.

The cure of disease is only possible when you eliminate the root of the problem. Some conditions in elderly animals may not be totally curable due to their shorter lifespans and the longstanding gravity of their conditions. With severely damaged organs, the homeopathic remedies still work on all the various levels, extending the quality and quantity of life, long beyond that which conventional medicine can usually provide.

There are thousands of different homeopathic remedies. These remedies are basically energy taken from natural substances such as plants and minerals. Every substance has an energetic blueprint: this is the basis of quantum physics, familiar to us with Einstein's famous equation: $E = mc2$, which proves that energy and mass are interchangeable.

When you administer the correct remedy, there is inevitably evidence of an incredible feeling of well-being. My clients will say, "Sparky is his old self again; he is acting like a puppy! He is doing all these things I haven't seen him do in years: getting in the garbage, climbing on the couch, chasing squirrels …" This is the result of the release of energy in the body that has been stuck in diseased energy patterns for so long. When this release occurs, there is a tremendous surge of vibrancy. How different from the side effects of conventional medicine that we are so familiar with—be it the debilitating effects of chemotherapy or the excessive water drinking, urinating or worse that accompany the administration of corticosteroids, just to name a few. No more of all those side effects and warnings listed in the pamphlets accompanying those drugs!

The only 'side effect', I tell my clients, is that their dogs will be happier and stronger, even in areas I may not know about, because it is the dog that I am treating, not the symptoms. This is particularly important in geriatric dogs, who are weaker and, therefore, much more sensitive and vulnerable to the ramifications of treatment with conventional drugs.

I have been using homeopathy for the past seventeen years and have treated thousands of dogs (and other animals). I would like to share a few of my cases. Happily, these examples are not unusual, they are typical of the 'miraculous' results that we can see using this energy modality. Every case is unique, however, and the story of these three dogs, are among my favorites. One of the most important keys to this kind of success story is, however, possibly a leap of faith and good owner compliance: Enjoy!

Mimosa

Mimosa was quite a character. A seven-year-old, female West Highland White Terrier, she first came to me accompanied by her guardian, Nicole. She had recently received a dire prognosis: she had been diagnosed with advanced kidney and liver failure and was given a month to live, both by her regular veterinarian and the board-certified neurologist from the referral hospital. Nicole had sought veterinary help because her canine friend had developed seizures. She was told that Mimosa's immune system was severely compromised and that she would shortly die of general organ failure. Despite the daily subcutaneous fluid therapy and the two medicines prescribed, her condition was deteriorating rapidly.

Not wanting to give up on her beloved dog, Nicole quickly called for an appointment when she heard about my homeopathic practice from a friend. Nicole was very familiar with homeopathy, as both she and her family had used it for themselves successfully in the past, and she was hopeful it could help her dog.

I remember well our initial consultation. Although the conventional diagnosis seemed grim and the blood work was concerning, Mimosa in no way looked like a dying dog to me. She had quite a strong vital force and was a tough, determined little girl who knew her mind; this dog did not want to die. I felt very confident that with good holistic care, Mimosa would improve. I switched her food immediately from a low-grade commercial diet to a raw, homemade one, stopped the drugs that I felt were harming rather than enhancing the function of her kidneys and liver, and started her on a homeopathic regime along with carefully selected nutritional supplements to support her failing organs.

The first remedy that I prescribed was *Nux Vomica*, which is derived from the seeds of an Asian tree. It is a clearing remedy that can help the body detoxify from the ill effects of drugs, which I felt were part of the presenting symptom picture. It is also of great use for the toxicity caused by kidney and liver failure. The mental picture is of a strong type A personality, which is what I felt Mimosa was despite her weakened state.

Each remedy has both a mental and a physical state, and because homeopathy follows the dictum of "like treats like", it is important that both the mental and physical state or symptoms of the patients match that of the remedy. Mimosa responded immediately, Nicole reported happily at our follow-up appointment. She was her old mischievous self, full of energy, running around like a puppy again. The new blood work, although not yet completely normal, was dramatically better. They began to call Mimosa the "miracle dog" at the local dog run.

As time went on, I treated Mimosa for many other issues. When she was ten years old, she presented a new challenge. Like so many New York City dogs, Mimosa had both a city and a country home. And like so many of them, she would get depressed when she returned to New York. Life was just more fun chasing squirrels and running on the beach rather than being leashed and walking on the sidewalk. Being the stubborn, willful little creature that she was, Mimosa took it a step further: she became moody and withdrawn, refusing to even look at her owner, angry and sulky that she wasn't getting her way and staying in the Hamptons. She put on weight, refused to budge and brooded. 'Indifference to those loved best' is that state described in the *Materia Medica*, or the book which is the compilation of all known homeopathic remedies, in which you do not show the love you truly feel for your beloved. This is a key indication for the use of *Sepia*, a homeopathic remedy made from the ink of the cuttlefish. This striking symptom, now evidenced by Mimosa's behavior toward Nicole, combined with her low energy, increase in weight and general apathy, confirmed my remedy selection, and, indeed, with it Mimosa returned to her usual high spirits, despite being back in the Big Apple.

At eleven-years-old, while running on the beach, Mimosa tore her anterior cruciate ligament. This is a knee injury that veterinarians see relatively often in dogs. Although the orthopedic surgeon insisted that the dog needed surgery to repair the leg, again, homeopathy came to the rescue. I would say that about 80 percent of my patients with torn ACL ligaments respond to homeopathy and do not need surgery. Many of them heal with the remedy Calcarea *Carbonica*, a substance derived from the inside of an oyster shell. It is a remedy with a particularly strong affinity for bone and joint issues, including weakness of ligaments and inflammation of the knee. Given the typically stubborn disposition of the patient who needs this remedy, I felt it fit the case, both mentally and physically. Within a few short weeks, Mimosa was as good as new.

At twelve, Mimosa started to slow down, and she settled into the sweet mellowness of older age. During these years, she developed a myriad of minor issues, such as crystals in the urine, ear and eye infections, even Lyme Disease, all of which I was able to treat homeopathically. But at fifteen and a half, she began to show serious signs of aging, and Nicole was becoming desperate thinking about how she would live without her best buddy, the longest and best relationship she has ever had, she told me—a comment that I often hear! "My friends are so worried about me," Nicole said. "How will I ever go on without little Mimosa?" So in preparation for the inevitable, Nicole acquired an adorable Yorkie puppy she named Missy. As is typical, the new puppy immediately adored her older 'sister,' but Mimosa seemed to pay her no need. Indeed, at sixteen she was virtually blind and deaf, and when I saw her in December, I knew it was time that she move on to the next plane. She had been given a death sentence at seven and was now sixteen, having lived an extra nine fabulous years, but the body cannot go on forever. It was time. Nicole had known that in her heart for a while now, but like many owners, needed the confirmation from her trusted veterinarian.

Nicole told me that in the taxi on the way home from my office, she set up an appointment for the house-call vet to euthanize Mimosa the following day. What she related to me next put a chill up my spine and brought tears to my eyes. The next morning, Mimosa grabbed her beloved stuffed animal—the one she couldn't be without for even one day of her life, the one Nicole had to have FedExed to the country when she forgot it one weekend, the one even Nicole wasn't allowed to touch, the one Mimosa had not played with for weeks. Mimosa took that toy and ran from room to room and, completing the tour around the apartment, dropped it at Missy's feet. Mimosa then retired to her bed and waited for the vet to come. She knew, and she was ready. After Mimosa's peaceful passing, Missy took the heretofore-untouched toy and immediately started playing with it. Mimosa died ten days after the arrival of Missy, whose presence, it seemed, gave her permission to leave. She knew how difficult it would be for her beloved mistress to be alone, and she had waited.

The baton had been passed.

Rajah

Rajah, a thin eleven-year-old shepherd/husky mix, stumbled into my Connecticut office one cold December day. Her back end was giving out, as it often does in so many other older, large breed dogs, and her guardian, Donatella, was terrified that her beloved companion would not make it to twelve. The dog was reluctant to move due to the painful arthritis that had developed in her dysplastic hips, and the nerve inflammation and degeneration in her spine was causing her back legs to shake and cross. She was tripping and falling more and more often. With my conventional hat on, I would have found this scenario heartbreaking, because without the benefit of alternative care, this presentation would often finish shortly in euthanasia. Happily, I was able to inform Donatella that this was not a life-threatening disease; this was merely a structural problem. Hopefully, I continued, Rajah could live for many more quality-filled years.

I began my homeopathic intake, as I normally do, with a strong emphasis on the dog's emotional and mental history, starting from when the client first acquired the dog. Homeopathy has the understanding, only now just beginning to be brought to light in the conventional realm, which is that most disease begins in the mind. It seems that Rajah had a very sad beginning. She was purchased by a young girl, eighteen years old, from a pet store. Just how long that little puppy had been in the tiny cage alone, Donatella could not be sure, but she did know, however, exactly how Rajah had spent those first months after leaving the pet store, as she was fortunate enough to have met the first owner, whom we shall call Alice. It seems that Alice was not a bad person, just ignorant about owning a dog. In fact, she wasn't even allowed to have a dog in the first place, as she was renting and the landlord forbid animals. Therefore, from three to six months of age, Rajah was kept chained in the basement. She subsequently, was forced to give the dog away. Rajah was ultimately passed around twice more before she ended up in a shelter, and all this before eight months of age.

Donatella was the director of therapeutic recreation and the volunteer coordinator for a nursing home. That facility had suggested she use a therapy dog for the residents, and that, coupled with her longstanding desire for a dog, was one lucky break for Rajah. It became her fourth and final home, and a winning situation on all fronts. So many of the elderly in nursing facilities lose their interest in living and often don't even want to leave their room. It has been found that therapy dogs brought into the facility, can stimulate their interest in life again and the desire for inter-action with the other residents, as well as with the dog.

Rajah became a stunning success story at the home, and their mascot. She would walk the corridors with Zipper the Cockatiel on her shoulder, and patiently and gently pull the wheelchairs, with the residents happily holding the other end of the leash. Thanks to Rajah, most of them would now participate in the recreation room events as well as in other activities. However, as considerate and compassionate as she was with the weak and vulnerable, Rajah would become a frightening demon when confronted by a five foot, six inch man with a beard, apparently her second home, where she was severely abused. Whenever, Rajah felt threatened, be it in a veterinarian's office or by a frightening figure to her, Rajah would use her snarl and her teeth, the only defense a dog really has, to keep the danger at bay. Almost all aggression, in fact, is due to fear.

Once finished with the mental and emotional history, I delve into the physical ailments of the dog. It seems Rajah had been hit by a car, while just a pup, evidenced by X-rays that Donatella had requested when her new dog showed lameness even as a youngster. The dog had done ad-equately for a while on some glucosamine supplements, but Donatella was now reluctant to put her dog on the strong anti-inflammatory drugs that her conventional veterinarian prescribed recently, as Rajah had already shown severe side effects to drugs in the past. And although the dog was strong and healthy in every other way, she didn't want to risk the damaging effects that the medicines could have. Familiar with the benefits of holistic medicine for herself and her family, she wanted the same kind of care for her canine companion.

I then addressed the present state of the dog and was concerned at her wasted frame, "Why is she so thin? Does she have an appetite?" I asked. "Oh yes," the attractive, middle-aged woman replied. "The vet told me to have her lose weight so as not to put more stress on the hips. She has already lost twenty pounds and has another ten to go." "Yes," I told her, "it is a good thing not to be overweight, but this dog is starving!"

It seemed she had been a healthy, 80-pound dog who was now emaciated at 60, and I shuddered to think what she would look like at 50. Gratefully, Donatella agreed, as she had been feeling so sorry for Rajah, who seemed hungry all the time.

This wonderful woman has long since become a dear friend of mine. She confessed to me that she felt she had come home as soon as she came into my office. She trusted me, observing that I was evaluating the whole dog, not just giving injections and pills that were potentially toxic and merely masking the pain. She appreciated being made part of the team. I had told her, as I tell all my patients, that it takes all of us to build the dog up to its maximum health: guardian, animal and doctor alike, we must all work together. As we embark on the path to better health, I teach the basics of homeopathy to guardians, recommend reading material, and have them keep a journal so they can monitor their dog's progress.

Rajah seemed a perfect candidate for acupuncture. Both the slipped discs and the hip dysplasia usually respond beautifully to it. However, when a dog enters my office with its own muzzle, as Rajah did, I know we may be in trouble. With muzzle in place, we gave it a try, but Rajah was terrified of veterinarians and needles, and shortly we knew that the dog had won this battle. "Not to worry," I told Donatella. This is one of the reasons I studied homeopathy: not all dogs, and certainly not all cats, are particularly fond of having needles inserted into their bodies, and so I wanted an alternative. What I found in homeopathy was an even deeper means of healing disease.

The first remedy I chose was *Lycopodium clavatum*, a treatment derived from a type of moss. Rajah's mental and emotional symptoms were a good match for those covered by the remedy. She exhibited a lack of confidence and apprehensiveness for which she over-compensated with a type of haughtiness or bossiness. Rajah was also a very jealous dog, coveting her owner's attention and becoming quite angry if her mistress deigned to pet another. On the physical level, she also showed the typical symptoms: lots of pain and weakness in the legs. In her case, the right leg was the worst. She even had the cracked and ulcerated occasionally bleeding nose often present when the patient needs *Lycopodium*. Since the basis of homeopathy is the law of similars, or "like treats like", I felt it was a good match physically, emotionally and mentally. Indeed, Rajah's follow-up report two weeks later showed that she was happier and much less stiff. She was not crossing her legs as often, was not 'bunny-hopping' any more (a sign of pain in the hips), and was not restlessly trying to find a comfortable position at night.

Over the course of the next four years, I treated Rajah with a series of various remedies. There was, as is often the case, a bit of a trial and error until we found the perfect fit, but with regular follow-ups and good owner compliance, "miracles" can happen. As Rajah aged, she developed a constitution more suited to *Causticum*, a remedy derived from Potassium Hydrate, that is often used for "broken down seniles." This is an old-fashioned term, used often in the Nineteenth and early Twentieth Century found in both the *Materia Medica*, and the *Reparatory*, which is an index of disease symptoms with the related remedies that can cure those symptoms.

"Broken down seniles" basically refers to geriatric individuals, whose bodies are deteriorating with age. *Causticum* is excellent for chronic arthritic and paralytic conditions, in which pain and deformities in the joints, along with progressive loss of muscular strength, gradually result in paralysis. Whenever I had hit upon the correct remedy with Rajah, inevitably I wrote "happier" in my notes. Seeing that sense of well-being in a dog I am treating is essential to know I am on the right track. With the aid of the remedies, Rajah mellowed into a more confident, well-adjusted dog who became the meeter and greeter at the dog park, a welcome change from the fearful, aggressive posturing she had carried with her from her earlier abuse. Her tail was no longer clenched tightly between her legs, as on her first visit, but was happily wagging.

Donatella told me over and over that she was very grateful that I had explained to her how homeopathy works and what to do in an emergency, because every so often, Rajah would slip and fall, either on the ice outside or on the wooden floors in the house. A dose or two of Arnica, the remedy par excellence for soft tissue injury, or *Hypericum*, the homeopathic derivation of *St. John's Wort* and the best remedy for nerve trauma, would put her on track, and she could avoid a trip to the emergency hospital when this scary situation occurred after hours.

Rajah lived happily and muzzle-free to the ripe old age of sixteen.

Rorie

Rorie, an eight-year-old Neapolitan Mastiff, hobbled into my office one sunny May day, walking on three legs, the left hind limb barely skimming the ground. The cause of the limp, Judy and Joan told me, was bone cancer. They showed me the radiograph, and I could see that the osteosarcoma was significantly advanced. In fact, the women told me, their vet had given Rorie no more than three months to live at best, whether or not they amputated the leg. The owners decided to see if there were any holistic options.

Given the advanced state of the tumor, I honestly did not know how much longer I could help the dog, especially because once the bone fractured, which it inevitably would, the dog would be in such severe pain that euthanasia would be the only option. I have extended the life of some dogs with bone cancer for even three years, but their cancer was not as advanced at presentation. Homeopathy can work extremely well with cancer, most of the time putting it into a remission where it does not progress or grows very slowly, possibly for years. The conventional veterinarian had put the dog on carprofen for pain, and although it seemed to help to some degree, the effects wore off rather quickly, and it broke Joan and Judy's hearts to see their dear friend becoming depressed, not wanting to move and whimpering in between doses. They, like most dog owners, did not want their dog to suffer, and with the grim diagnosis, it didn't make sense to keep her going if she would have to live out her days like this.

Emotionally, Rorie was a very nurturing dog, always caring for and protecting her owners, as if they were her own children. Usually, owners take care of their animal friends, Joan and Judy told me, but Rorie was the only dog that they'd ever had who they felt was taking care of them. These grey giants were indeed bred for protection, but this was beyond the call of duty. In contrast to her imposing form, she had an extremely sweet disposition, and when she was in pain, unlike so many other dogs who become irritable and withdrawn, she sought the comfort and affection of her owners, which was out of character for her. The pain in her leg was worse with movement and seemed to come on suddenly and violently. These symptoms are often treated with the homeopathic remedy *Pulsatilla nigricans*, which is made from the wind flower.

Based on her emotional, mental and physical symptoms, I chose to administer this remedy. Pulsatilla, in varying strengths, carried Rorie through the next six months. Immediately on her initial two-week follow up, Joan and Judy reported to me that the dog felt better. She no longer craved extra attention, would happily move around the house and go for short walks. There was absolutely no more need for the anti-inflammatory drug, for she was her old self. The remedy would wear off every month or two and need to be repeated in ascending doses, but Rorie would never, for the rest of her life, manifest any of the terrible pain that she felt prior to and in between doses of the carprofen. Her owners would know when she needed another dose when she sought more attention, which indicated only some mild discomfort. No more of the crying, whimpering and reluctance to move was experienced, pre-carprofen.

Because the family lived three hours away from me, most of the follow-up after the first consultation was done via phone calls. But six months later, the owners called me to say that they thought I should see their dog, even though she was happy and eating and walking. When they showed up at my office, my mouth literally hung open. The dog's leg was tremendously swollen, almost like elephantiasis, but the dog didn't seem to notice. She was a happy girl, walking on her own, and at 120 pounds, she truly had to! I found it incredible that the mastiff felt absolutely no pain at all. The leg had obviously fractured, probably some months ago, but that didn't seem to put even a dent in her good mood.

Rorie was a fighter who never gave up: even now, they told me, she would insist on going up the stairs to the bedroom every night, and into the car for rides. One of them would assist with her hindquarters, but Rorie was doing most of the work. Joan and Judy realized how bad the leg looked, but they told me they just couldn't put her down because she was happy and, except for some difficulty in dragging that leg along, seemed totally normal.

A few days later, I received a happy, excited phone call. Rorie had passed. "What happened?" I asked. "Well, it was just incredible," Joan reported. Rorie had woken up and, just like any other morning, devoured her big bowl of homemade food, then let out a deep, satisfied sigh and died. Unable to believe what they had witnessed, they kept checking her to make sure she really was dead. Of course, they were very saddened to have lost their best friend, they said, but what a way to go!

These examples demonstrate the power of homeopathy. Be aware that it is a difficult and complex system of medicine to master, and it can take years for a practitioner to become proficient enough to treat the chronic diseases that we see so often in geriatric dogs.

> *It is always best for a pet owner to consult with a veterinary homeopath, rather than to try to treat the advanced pathology of chronic disease of their pet on their own.*

In the United States, there is one national organization for veterinary homeopaths, which is the Academy of Veterinary Homeopathy (*www.TheAVH.org*). This organization, which has a rigorous training program and sets extremely high standards of practice, is an excellent resource for finding a competent homeopath for your dog. I completed many years of additional training in England where there is also an excellent British organization, the British Academy of Veterinary Homeopaths, (*www.BAVHS.org*), where pet owners can research a competent veterinary homeopath. There are training programs for homeopaths all around the world, and it is best to look into the educational background of a practitioner, before selecting one for your pet. However, as is true with conventional doctors, it is not just the years in practice that counts, oftentimes, novices make up in enthusiasm and determination, with what they lack in actual experience. And, as is true with any profession, referrals, in this case from happy dog owners, is invaluable.

It can, however, be extremely easy and simple to treat many acute injuries and conditions with one of the many good reference books written specifically for the pet owner. A few of my favorite homeopathic books are listed below. However, more and more informative works for the pet owner are finding their way onto the shelves at your local bookstore or online. On a personal note, one of my greatest gratifications, is when I am asked to refer my clients to a homeopath who treats humans, as they say their dog is going to outlive them, they are doing so well!

Marcie Fallek, DVM, CVA is a Holistic Veterinarian Specializing in Classical Homeopathy with offices in Manhattan and Connecticut. She is the National Representative of the United States of America to the International Academy of Veterinary Homeopathy (IAVH). She has her B.A. in Philosophy and Literature from Boston University and her DVM from the University of Bologna, Italy. She is also certified in veterinary acupuncture. Dr Fallek trained initially with Dr. Richard Pitcairn, completing both the basic and advanced training levels She then went on to study for many years in the U.K., first with the Orion School in London and then completed a five year course and three years of post graduate training with the Homeopathic Physicians Teaching Group in Oxford, England, a specialized training program for Medical

Doctors and Veterinarians. She is on the board of the IAVH and is a member of the American Holistic Veterinary Medical Association as well as many others.

148 E 40th Street, New York, NY 10016
248 Alden Street, Fairfield, CT 06824
212-216-9177
www.Holisticvet.us
Marciefallek@earthlink.net

My Favorite Resources:

Dr. Pitcairn's Complete Guide to Natural Health for Dogs and Cats
     by Pitcairn, Richard
Homeopathic Care for Cats and Dogs by Hamilton, Don
Homeopathic First Aid for Animals by Walker, Kaetheryn
The Academy of Veterinary Homeopathy
     www.TheAVH.org

17

Quality of Life
by Alice E. Villalobos, DVM, DPNAP

How do I care for my dog at the end of life stage?

How will I know when it is the right time to make the final call for the gift of euthanasia?

The Human-Animal bond embraces love and respect for owner and pet in society. People are emotionally shocked when their beloved pet is diagnosed with life-limiting or advanced stages of disease. Pet lovers are demanding that veterinarians step up to provide more comprehensive end of life services for their pets as long as the pet is able to maintain a good quality of life (QoL).

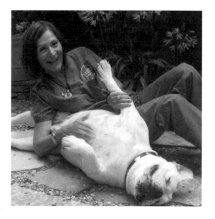

Veterinarians typically don't know about or avoid the challenges that come with end of life care. Why is that? Many veterinarians say that they are obligated to prevent and relieve animal suffering and they feel that end of life care drags out the inevitable.

This might sound insensitive to many readers of this book, but most veterinarians try to do what they feel is right. It might be that until recently, veterinary education focused on only three stages of life: the puppy and kitten stage, the adult stage and the senior stage. There is a true "Fourth Stage of Life" that has been bypassed, yet it might last for quite a while. That fourth stage of life, which the love and tenacity within the human-animal bond will no longer bypass, is "The End of Life Stage." Since it is all about QoL, how can one evaluate, measure or define QoL?

Society accepts that humane euthanasia (well, death) for companion animals is indeed the best option when QoL is lost or the best way to mercifully end pointless suffering. This viewpoint may have served the veterinary profession and society adequately in the past. But today, pet lovers want more options when their pets are aging or are diagnosed with life-limiting disease or cancer.

> *Modern pain management, high tech medicine and good nursing care can restore and maintain QoL for longer periods. Caregivers want to extend the timeline between the diagnosis of a terminal disease and death for their companion animals.*

Society's wish to provide end of life care for companion animals raises lots of bioethical questions such as:

- What are one's obligations to their companion animal?

- Must all of the disorders in my companion animals be addressed?

- Is palliative care (treating symptoms without intent to cure) good enough?

- How can one evaluate or assess an animal's QoL?

- How can one restore and maintain QoL?

- How will I know when it is the right time to make the final call for the gift of euthanasia?

- What if my religious or personal beliefs about my animals are not in alignment with my community?

All pet caregivers have an obligation to properly assess their pets' QoL and to maintain the best quality of life for their animals as possible. Society agrees that people have an obligation to confront the issues that ruin the QoL of their animals such as: cruelty, starvation, dehydration, confinement, untreated and undiagnosed suffering and neglect. These issues and an animal's needs are particularly important when families are caring for aging, ailing or terminally ill pets.

Veterinarians are frequently asked to treat symptoms in their animal patients without the aid of diagnostic tests. This is actually palliative care which treats a given set of symptoms based upon the doctor's best professional guess. It is seldom explained as palliative care to their clients, but it is. Human medical physicians shifted away from palliative care thinking that they "can do" something no matter what the cost or the side effects would be.

Physicians felt like failures if they chose palliation or hospice because they were taught to never give up. Unfortunately, millions of people undergo high risk treatments at the end of life. This often causes adverse effects. Denied the option for palliative care, many patients die poorly in hospitals or intensive care wards instead of dying peacefully with home hospice, surrounded by their families and friends.

It will take time for the entire veterinary profession to embrace palliative care, hospice and/or Pawspice care. Pawspice includes treating symptoms and primary disease with kinder, gentler standard care and transitions to hospice as the animal nears death. Pawspice may start early, when a pet is diagnosed with a life-limiting disease. QoL is the goal for all who care for pets with life-limiting disease. Unfortunately, very little work has been published in assessing QoL at the end of an animal's life. For this reason, pet owners must rely on the experience of veterinary caregivers worldwide and this author's forty plus years of experience. Combined, this group has cared for millions of animal cancer patients, including this author who has escorted thousands of beloved companion animals to the very end of their lives.

The "HHHHHHMM" Quality of Life Scale

Alice Villalobos, DVM, DPNAP, a renowned veterinary oncologist, introduced "Pawspice", a quality of life program based on a Quality of Life Scale for companion animals with terminal disease. Pawspice (rhymes with hospice) starts at diagnosis of a life limiting condition. It addresses cancer with kinder gentler standard care, embraces palliative management for uncomfortable symptoms, and transitions into hospice (more intense care) as the patient declines toward death. *The HHHHHMM Quality of Life Scale* provides a scoring system of 0-10 for family members and veterinary teams to assess a pet's condition during Pawspice. The Acronym's five **H**'s stand for: *H*urt, *H*unger, *H*ydration, *H*ygiene and *H*appiness. The two **M**'s stand for *M*obility and *M*ore good days than bad days. The QoL scale is also a decision making tool for family to face their responsibilities and prevent suffering with the gift of euthanasia to assure that their sick animal has a peaceful and painless passing. Download at *www.pawspice.com.*

Table 1.
Quality of Life Scale
(The HHHHHMM Scale)

Caregivers can use this Quality of Life Scale to assess animals and guide decision making for Pawspice care. Use numbers from 0 to 10 (10 is ideal or normal) to score the patient's condition.	
Score	**Criterion**
0-10	**HURT** - Adequate pain control & breathing ability is top priority. Trouble breathing outweighs all concerns. Is pain being treated properly or not? Can the animal breathe properly? Is supplemental oxygen necessary?
0-10	**HUNGER** - Is the pet eating enough? Does hand feeding help? Does the patient need a feeding tube?

0-10	**HYDRATION** - Is the pet dehydrated? For patients not drinking enough water, use subcutaneous fluids daily or twice daily to supplement fluid intake.
0-10	**HYGIENE** - The pet should be brushed and cleaned, particularly after eliminations. Avoid pressure sores with soft bedding and keep all wounds clean.
0-10	**HAPPINESS** - Does the pet express joy and interest? Is the pet responsive to family, toys, etc.? Is the pet depressed, lonely, anxious, bored or afraid? Can the pet's bed be moved to be close to family activities?
0-10	**MOBILITY** - Can the pet get up without assistance? Does the pet need human or mechanical help? Is the dog willing/able to go out for short walks? Is the pet having seizures or stumbling? Some feel euthanasia is preferable to amputation. But a companion animal with 3 legs or limited mobility can be alert, happy and have a very good QoL only if the family is committed to helping their companion animal get around with: ramps, cart, harness, braces, rehab., acupunct., etc.
0-10	**MORE GOOD DAYS THAN BAD** - When bad days outnumber good days, QoL may be too compromised. When a healthy human-animal bond is no longer possible, the family must be made aware that the end is near. The decision for euthanasia needs to be made if the animal has pointless suffering. If death comes peacefully and painlessly at home, that is okay.
*TOTAL	*A total over 35 points represents acceptable life quality to continue with Pawspice/hospice.

Original concept, *Oncology Outlook*, by Dr. Alice Villalobos, *Quality of Life Scale Helps Make Final Call*, VPN, 09/2004; scale format created for author's textbook, *Canine and Feline Geriatric Oncoloty: Honoring the Human-Animal Bond*, Blackwell Pub., 2007. Adapted for CB, VCNA, AAFP, IVAPM's *Palliative Care & Hospice Statement, Senior Dog Books & Merial's pre-VCS/ESVONC/ WVCC-RT, 2012,* with permission from Dr. Villalobos & Wiley

Just as in older people, older pets have one or more conditions that bother them. How do we know when a chronic, comorbid condition starts to ruin a pet's QoL?

> *The most common conditions affecting older dogs and cats are: dental disease, painful arthritis, obesity and various disorders related to organ disease and organ failure.*

If an older dog is diagnosed with a life-limiting disease or cancer, its related treatment will add more burdens on the already compromised animal. It is important to determine if the pet's QoL will be impacted by the disease and the recommended treatment.

What is the risk-benefit ratio of the treatment?

Who is capable of properly monitoring the patient?

How are they making their decisions?

At what point should caregivers abandon further curative therapy?

Veterinarians are frequently asked, "When is the right time to euthanize my beloved pet? How will I know?" People look for answers to these difficult questions from Dr. Internet. They often find too much unreliable information and extensive marketing for remedies with amazing claims or promises. It is best to search for the disease by its name and species (dog, cat, ferret, horse, etc.) and add the words, "veterinary college" to get reliable information. People often browse the Internet for decision aids while their attending doctors might be unaware [2].

Respect Needs and Desires

Animals have certain needs and desires which should be recognized and respected by their caretakers. The Five Freedoms of Animal Welfare was developed for farm animals in the United Kingdom. Yet this list is useable for all companion animals. The Five Freedoms from the Farm Animals Welfare Council are:

1. Freedom from Hunger and Thirst
2. Freedom from Discomfort
3. Freedom from Pain, Injury or Disease
4. Freedom to Express Normal Behavior
5. Freedom from Fear and Distress

If one is able to maintain the five basic needs and desires during end of life care, then there is justification for pet owners to care for their failing pets with palliative care programs and Pawspice or hospice. The QoL Scale helps animal caregivers to confidently determine what a satisfactory QoL should be.

The *HHHHHMM QoL Scale* above provides useful guidelines for caregivers to help sustain a positive and rewarding relationship that nurtures the human-animal bond at the end of life. This simple to use tool helps pet owners discuss issues with their veterinarian during exam room visits. The QoL Scale provides a framework to assess various aspects of home care and patient well being. The straightforward QoL Scale, with its objective scoring, automatically helps family members face reality without guilt feelings or confusion. The QoL Scale asks people to score their observations on a scale of 0-10 with 10 being the best or normal. It helps each family member struggle through the difficult decision making process of whether to maintain their beloved pet in further decline or to elect the gift of euthanasia.

If family members are able to correct deficient criteria by at least 30 to 60 percent, improvements might create a remarkable rejuvenation in a failing pet's well being. Ask the veterinary team for help. They are experts in teaching how to assess and control pain. They often teach their clients how to provide good nutritional and hydration support for general medicine patients. When discussing hygiene, the nursing staff can demonstrate wound care techniques and ways to prevent bed sores (decubitus ulcers) by using egg crate mattresses, soft bedding and body rotation. The nursing staff can show pet lovers how to keep their pets cleaner and to prevent self-soiling using elevation mats, absorbent towels, diapers and so forth.

> *The QoL Scale helps families realize that they might need to ratchet up certain aspects of their home care program to properly maintain their pet more comfortably. A well-managed end of life care program using palliative care (symptom treatment), Pawspice or hospice allows more quality time for the human-animal bond. Tender private moments and sweet conversations are shared between family members and their beloved pet during the bumpy road toward death.*

Acute vs. Chronic Hospitalization at End of Life

The most important QoL factors to monitor are: pain, respiration, blood flow, maintaining adequate nutrition, hydration and temperature. Factors to avoid are depression and frustration. Most experts agree that it is in the animal's best interest to be at home with familiar, consistent routine and surroundings [3].

How long should a sick or dying animal remain in the hospital? Hospitalized pets are susceptible to the same "hospitalism" syndrome (failure to thrive) that infants and geriatric people acquire when they are hospitalized for long periods. Hospitalism occurs because infants and geriatric patients are only handled when wet, being fed or medicated. Efforts to avoid hospitalism for end of life pets are justified. This would include considering the hospice option for companion animals that are taken to emergency clinics in subacute and acute terminal crisis conditions.

A common example would be dogs with hemoabdomen (blood in the belly). Dogs develop tumors in the spleen or liver made of blood vessel wall cells (hemangiosarcoma) that often rupture. It is estimated that two million dogs will die of this cancer. A large percentage are reluctantly euthanized in the "either or" medicine model after triage at local emergency clinics. If surgery is declined due to the poor prognosis or financial constraints, hospice should be a third option. Upset pet owners feel rushed and pushed to euthanize their pet in the either or model.

If the family wants more time, patients can and should be released, with a signed consent form, to go home with steroids, pain medication and a belly wrap. This gives an opportunity for the home hospice vigil and home euthanasia. Occasionally, red blood cells are resorbed and some dogs might rally for a week or two and provide their families with a more extended farewell. One such dog actually survived an amazing nine months with good QoL. The family documented five episodes of bleeding that required belly wraps and rest.

Patient Criteria to Score and Improve

No Hurt: pain assessment techniques

Millions of companion animals suffer in silence without their families recognizing it. Animals do not exhibit pain the way that people do. To prevent animal suffering, people need to recognize it. Pain assessment aids and questionnaires may yield variable results due to owner ignorance, inexperience, insensitivity and bias. Veterinarians are highly trained to assess for all types of pain during the physical examination. They will ask questions and educate pet owners to look for signs of pain [4].

The horrible and desperate pain of respiratory distress ranks at the top for humans and it is presumed to be the same for animals. Not being able to breathe outweighs all other criteria. Respiratory distress is an emergency and it must be relieved immediately or there is no QoL for the animal and there is no humane justification to continue the hospice.

Human cancer patients often feel their pain more resoundingly at night and it seems to be true for animal cancer patients as well. Cancer pain has multiple pathways—it involves stimulation of pain receptors, tissue damage, inflammation, peripheral and central sensitization and wind up pain. Superficial attempts at cancer pain management are generally not enough to restore QoL. Cancer pain most often requires combination therapy tailored to the patient's condition and organ function. If in doubt, pain therapy should be given for at least a few days or a week to observe if the animal feels better, moves around more and sleeps better.

Cancer pain, arthritis pain or muscle pain may respond to one or a combination of agents such as: drugs, nutraceuticals, physical (rehabilitation) therapy and complementary medicine techniques such as massage, acupuncture, chiropractic, low level laser therapy, and low level sonic vertical vibration therapy, etc. The International Veterinary Association of Pain Management (IVAPM) has advocated pain management education to veterinarians. It is an extensive topic with recent board certification. Pain management is discussed in greater detail in many other resources.[5, 6].

No Hunger: Poor Appetite and Poor Nutrition

Weight loss can be sneaky under the beautiful coat that most companion animals were blessed with. Therefore monitoring an older or ill pet's weight is essential. Malnutrition, weight loss and cancer cachexia (extreme weight loss due to cancer) develop quickly in animals when their appetite is poor. Pet owners are not educated regarding minimum caloric intake or resting energy requirement (RER). The veterinarian can prescribe appetite stimulants such as mirtazapine. Along with coaxing, hand feeding or gentle force feeding with wholesome, flavorful foods, one might restore and maintain adequate nutritional intake for their failing pet.

If a dog or cat drops 10 percent of body weight and is not consuming its RER for three to five days, then feeding tube placement must be considered. This option prevents further weight loss and decline from malnutrition, dehydration and starvation while maintaining gut health.

Blended or liquid recovery diets will help maintain proper nutritional and caloric intake via the E-Tube. At times, attending doctors and pet owners are not in favor of the idea of placing feeding tubes for end of life care; however, the patient needs and requires adequate nutrition if a good QoL hospice is to continue. Companion animals are fortunate. They do not have to endure the ravages of anorexia, starvation, dehydration and unnecessary pain before death because society protects and sanctions innocent animals from pointless suffering. Society grants animals a peaceful and painless passing with the gift of euthanasia.

Every effort should be made to control nausea and vomiting which may be contributing to the pet's poor appetite and cause complete anorexia. Maropitant (Cerenia™) acts in the brain to reduce vomiting and nausea. Maropitant was also documented to provide significant abdominal pain control. This feature provides added comfort for palliative and hospice patients [7]. Reglan™ Anzemet™ and Zofran™ are also widely used to control or reduce vomiting. Pepcid and sucralfate may also be used to provide gastrointestinal comfort care.

Many pet lovers may not want or be able to afford standard medical treatments for their aging or ailing pets. They may prefer nutritional support in the form of immunonutrition as the only therapy for their pet. Ageing, illness, chronic stress and fatigue are known to lower the immune status of humans and animals. Aging and obesity is associated with chronic inflammation. These co-morbid conditions create a less efficient or altered immune response. This situation places the patient at a higher risk for infections, arthritis, endocrine disorders such as hypothyroidism, Cushing's disease and diabetes, autoimmune diseases and cancer.

Providing good nutrition and supplements for ill, geriatric and ambulatory end of life patients may benefit their innate immune system receptors. These receptors are located in the gut which is the largest immune organ in the body. Many pet owners are pleased with the QoL benefits which high quality targeted immunonutrition brings to their aging and ailing companion animals[8]. For more information see *Sensible Supplements* in the library section at www.Pawspice.com.

No Hydration Problems

Every companion animal being kept in end of life care should be given adequate fluid intake (two teaspoons or 10 ml per pound per day). The veterinarian can teach caregivers to assess their pet's hydration by the pinch method. If the pinched skin is slow to return to normal position, the animal is dehydrated. Giving subcutaneous (SQ) fluids at home is a wonderful way to supplement the fluid intake of ailing pets. This saves money and keeps the patient healthier with a huge improvement in QoL.

Good hygiene

Open, weeping, necrotic wounds may need professional help for debridement (cleaning away of dead tissue) and partial closure to promote healing. Chronic wounds may need bacterial culture and specific antibiotics. The modern principles of wound care have changed. Gentle cleaning with saline rinses or sprays, wound surfactants such as sugar can lift away bacteria without tissue damage. Moist bandages that promote healing can be very helpful [9].

Malignant wounds are very difficult to care for. Some large open tumors respond to palliative radiation therapy. Some animals need intense pain management to control haunting attacks of acute pain (allodynia). Many pets need protective bandages or stockinet to cover and protect bandages on their limbs. Some animals benefit greatly with body suits which are designed to help animals avoid self-mutilation.

Happiness: Serum Fun Factors

Not everyone agrees that an animal's QoL should include psychosocial well being. This author believes that a good Pawspice must include a two-way exchange of pleasure and contentment between the pet owner and the pet along with enrichment that encourages as much fun as possible. Happiness generates good physiology and mental well being and longer survival times[10]. It is important to create frequent moments of enjoyment for the ailing pet. Many end of life pets cheer up and look forward to these uplifting events. The beneficial effect of joy and happiness may be from increasing the "serum fun factors." Having fun during these special days can make a world of difference for family members and the patient.

The human pediatric cancer care model strives to entertain children with enjoyable programs and so does Pawspice. End of life pets need to derive some pleasure from being alive and some enjoyment (being petted and talked to) for a good part of their day and to have actual fun if at all possible. [11]. Ask these questions:

Does the pet express joy and show interest in the family?

Is the pet responsive to caressing and the environment?

Is the pet depressed, lonely, anxious, bored or afraid?

Is the pet isolated?

Can the pet's bed be moved near family activities and be in the middle of things?

Mobility: A Flexible Criterion

The answer to the mobility question has viable and variable scenarios. Utilitarian pet owners may be rigid in their mobility requirements for their dog(s). Some pet owners will euthanize their large dog rather than elect amputation of a limb for bone cancer. Some pet owners might unwittingly allow their bone cancer dog to bear a painful limb for months before electing the gift of euthanasia. Some pet owners and some cultures such as the Swedish feel that amputation for a companion animal is mutilation. They believe that amputation is not fair to the animal [12]. Of course there are many studies and testimonials and YouTube videos that show a good QoL for pets missing one and even two limbs. However, changing a person's viewpoint may be impossible even with knowledge and visual proof that a dog can lead a happy life without a limb.

Nursing care of immobile large dogs is very demanding and may be physically impossible for many pet owners to deal with. Ask yourself:

Can the dog be lifted up and taken outdoors for daily eliminations?

Will a harness, a sling or cart help?

Is medication helping?

Is there a schedule with family members willing to change the position and rotate the pet every two hours?

For animals that are immobile, care must be taken to avoid lung collapse (atelectasis) and bed sores (decubitus ulcers).

Is the bedding material soft enough?

Can an egg crate mattress be used and set up properly to avoid decubitus ulcers?

Will the pet benefit with a pet wheel chair, mobility cart or an Evans standing cart (*www.Jorvet.com*)?

These items can greatly facilitate keeping pets with limited mobility and allows them to experience more QoL with more joy and well being.

More Good Days than Bad Days

If a terminal pet experiences more than three to five bad days in a row, QoL is too compromised to continue the hospice. When a healthy, two-way interactive human-animal bond is no longer possible, it is time to let go. If the HHHHHMM QoL Score drops below 35, all family members will become aware that the end is near. The final decision needs to be made if the pet suffers breakthrough pain despite adjusting the pain medications.

> *The veterinary oath clearly obligates veterinarians to prevent animal suffering.*

It is best for the patient to be given heavy sedation to ease pain and anxiety before the kind gift of a bond-centered euthanasia. The euthanasia may be planned at home, at the local pet hospital or in the event of an afterhour's crisis, at a designated emergency clinic.

Do Not Allow Hospice Pets to Slowly Suffer to Death

Due to cultural, religious or personal beliefs, a few pet owners and a small contingent of veterinarians and counselors prefer "natural death" over assisted death. When a pet owner has this bias, it can be very difficult and disheartening for their attending veterinary team. They feel badly because they can't compromise their personal ethics. They can't justify caring for an emaciated, dehydrated, depressed terminal patient that must endure further deterioration, pointless pain and suffering until liberated by death.

When a veterinarian or pet hospice counselor has the natural death bias, it affects how they think and how they influence their client's decision making for a terminal pet when the bad days persist without any good days. The attending doctor or counselor may be sincerely attempting to respect the owner's wishes while caring for the patient, yet they may be totally unaware of how they are manipulating their clients into withholding the mercy of euthanasia for the dying pet, if or when it is needed. This is another version of the "either or" model mentioned above. By withholding options in the either or model, the attending doctors are practicing the strongest form of coercion [13].

It is considered ideal and fortunate if a companion animal is able to die at home with family in a painless and peaceful state. A peaceful and painless passing is most predictable when using veterinary supervision that includes proper pain control and home euthanasia services. Not all terminal animals receive professional help nor are they able to pass away peacefully and naturally at home. Some dying companion animals suffer greatly and go into horribly painful respiratory distress and thrash about and become agonal before death.

Slow dying is truly not natural for animals at all. In nature's way of the wild, debilitated animals naturally become prey. Sick animals in the wild do not survive long enough in decline to endure the angst of slowly suffering to death. Witnessing a beloved companion's active death can be a horrible experience for loving family members. They did not want their beloved pet to suffer pointless pain and indignity without having the option of humane euthanasia. Family members feel guilty and are haunted for years with these harsh memories.

Pet owners who prefer "natural death" need professional counseling to see if they are avoiding the responsibility to be their pet's protector. They should be the one who protects their pet from unnecessary suffering before death. If the reason for preferring natural death is religious or spiritual, they must still not allow their pet to suffer. They need to be educated on using the QoL scale to detect pain and discomfort and to provide adequate pain medication and comfort care all the way to the end. They should always have a backup plan in case their actively dying pet has a distressful crisis and needs professional help to change worlds. The contingency plan is rushing to an emergency clinic for the gift of euthanasia before allowing their innocent pet to suffer to death.

Framework for Ethical Decision Making

Download the *Framework for Ethical Decision Making* by going to (*www.Ethics.ubc.ca*) and clicking documents, then framework for ethical decision making. Mike McDonald's framework urges all involved parties, including attending doctors, specialists, hospital staff and the family, to reach consensus and comfort with their decisions, especially in their final decisions. When adapting this framework for animals, caregivers must prioritize the pet's best interests and QoL.

All veterinarians should offer palliative care or hospice or, better yet, Pawspice care for terminal animals embracing the family with a compassionate attitude. The more hopeful clients with ambulatory pets might prefer Pawspice care which combines palliative care with kinder, gentler versions of standard care and immunonutrition and transitions into hospice when the pet is expected to die within a few weeks [14]. There is no perfect choice, but the course taken should feel reasonably acceptable by those involved under the circumstances [15].

Summary

Companion animal lovers have an ethical obligation to maintain QoL as their pet ages and enter the newly recognized and unavoidable stage of life that is "End of Life." *The HHHHHMM QoL Scale* is a user friendly tool which directs caregivers to assess and score eight essential criteria for QoL on a monthly, weekly, daily or hourly basis as needed. The family can learn to conscientiously monitor and improve their failing pet's QoL score to maintain an acceptable well being which validates the human-animal bond.

Using the *Framework for Ethical Decision Making* can also help pet lovers make difficult decisions. End of life care focuses on QoL by adopting palliative care, hospice or Pawspice instead of curative treatment.

Focusing on QoL may be the best option for terminal patients to avoid "the mindless machinery of medicine" that so many human patients and their families are coerced into electing in the either or/can do medicine model [16].

Focusing on QoL for companion animals with life-limiting disease may avoid futile medicine, overtreatment and reluctant early euthanasia.

Focusing on QoL allows the human-animal bond to last longer. It allows terminal pets and their families to enjoy a celebrated new stage of life that truly is a distinct and loving journey at the end of life.

> *"Primum Non Nocere. First, do no harm."*
> *– Hippocrates*

Dr. Alice Villalobos is a pioneer in cancer care for pets. She completed a three year preliminary residency program in veterinary clinical oncology under the direction of Dr. Gordon H. Theilen and earned her doctorate from the UC Davis School of Veterinary Medicine in 1972. She was Founder and Director of Coast Pet Clinic/Animal Cancer Center, a multispecialty facility in Hermosa Beach, CA which provided an internship program, emergency and oncology services, including radiation therapy, to the greater Los Angeles area. After 24 years, Dr. Villalobos partnered her facility with Veterinary Centers of America. She is Director of Pawspice in Hermosa Beach and Animal Oncology Consultation Service in Woodland Hills, CA. Dr. Villalobos is a founding member of the Veterinary Cancer Society, the Association of Veterinary Family Practice and the International Association for Animal Hospice and Palliative Care.

She is President of the Society for Veterinary Medical Ethics (SVME), past president and editor-in-chief for the American Association of Human-Animal Bond Veterinarians (AAH-ABV) and a long time member of the AVMA, CVMA, SCVMA, AAHA, NAVC, VCS, AHF, SOPHIE and HSVMA. She is a Distinguished Practitioner of the

National Academies of Practice and serves as Chair of the Veterinary Academy. She is author of the textbook, Canine and Feline Geriatric Oncology: Honoring the Human-Animal Bond *(Blackwell Publishing, 2007) and "The Bond and Beyond", a column in Veterinary Practice News. In 1977, Dr. Villalobos Founded the Peter Zippi Memorial Fund for Animals which documents over 12,000 rescued animals. She is an honored recipient of the Leo Bustad Companion Animal Veterinarian Award and the UC Davis Alumni Achievement Award "for her pioneering role in bringing oncology services to companion animals." Dr. Villalobos writes and lectures worldwide on veterinary oncology, quality of life, bioethics, the human-animal bond and palliative/ hospice care for animals. She introduced the concept of "Pawspice" to the veterinary profession for end of life care and created a well known Quality of Life Scale to assess animal patients which may be downloaded at www.Pawspice.com. Pawspice (which rhymes with hospice) combines palliative care with kinder, gentler standard care for companion animals diagnosed with cancer and other life-limiting disease. Pawspice transitions into hospice care as the patient declines toward death.*

Pawspice at VCA Coast Animal Hospital, Hermosa Beach, CA and Animal Oncology Consultation Service, at Animal Emergency and Care Center, Woodland Hills, CA

President, Society for Veterinary Medical Ethics:
www.SVME.org
www.pawspice.com
dralicev@aol.com

My Favorite Resources:

Kaplan, Laurie (2011), *So Easy to Love, So Hard to Lose,* JanGen Press, Briarcliff, New York.

Kay, Nancy, (2010), *Speaking for Spot,* Trafalgar Square Books, North Pomfret, Vermont Sife, Wallace, Ph.D. (2005).

T*he Loss of a Pet, 3rd Ed.,* Howell Book House, Published by Wiley Publishing, Hoboken, New Jersey.

Villalobos A, Kaplan L, (2007), *Canine and Feline Geriatric Oncology: Honoring the Human-Animal Bond,* Blackwell Publishing, Ames, Iowa, (now Wiley Publishing, Hoboken, New Jersey).

Sife, Wallace, Ph.D. (2005) *The Loss of a Pet, 3rd Ed.,* Howell Book House.

Association for Pet Loss and Bereavement
www.aplb.org

Recommended Reading

1. Villalobos A, Kaplan L, Canine and Feline Geriatric Oncology: Honoring the Human-Animal Bond, Blackwell Publishing (Wiley-Blackwell), Hoboken, NY, 2007.

2. Brace C, *Journal of Clinical Oncology* (2010;28:2286-2292).

3. Stella JL, Lord LK, Buffington CA, Sickness behaviors in response to unusual external events in healthy cats and cats with feline interstitial cystitis, JAVMA, Vol. 238, No.1, 2011, p. 67-73.

4. Lascelles BDX, Supportive Care for the Cancer Patient, Ch. 16 in Small Animal Clinical Oncology, 4th Ed. Withrow & Vail, Saunders/Elsevier, 2007, p 291-346.

5. Gaynor JS, Muir WW, Handbook of Veterinary Pain Management, Mosby/Elsevier, 2008.

6. Jones K, et al, IVAPM Statement: Pain Management for End of Life Care, 2011.

7. Twedt D, Chronic Vomiting: a practical clinical approach, SVMA Syllalbus, 2011.

8. Satyaraj E, Immunonutrition, Nestle Purina Nutrition Forum: Changing Paradigms in Nutrition, St. Louis, MO, 2008.

9. Hendrickson, DA, Advanced Wound Care, SVMA Syllabus, 2011.

10. Rollin BE, Oncology and Ethics, AVMA Proceedings, 2004.

11. Rollin BE, Animal Happiness, A Philosophical View, Mental Health and Well Being in Animals, ed. McMillan, F.D., 2005, p235-242.

12. Yeates JW, Main DCJ, The ethics of influencing clients, Views: Commentary, JAVMA, Vol. 237, No. 3, August 1, 2010, p 263-267.

13. Voith VL, Attachment of People to Companion Animals, VCNA, Vol. 15, No. 2, The Human-Companion Animal Bond, March 1985, W.B. Saunders Company, Philadelphia PA, 1985.

14. Villalobos A. "Pawspice" an End of Life Care Program for Terminal Patients, Ch. 16b, Withrow, McEwen & Vail, Small Animal Clinical Oncology, 4th Ed., W.B. Saunders, Philadelphia PA, 2007.

15. McDonald, M, An ethical decision making framework. (Unpublished Document), University of British Columbia Centre for Applied Ethics, 2002, http://www.ethics.ubc.ca.

16. Temel, J.S., Early Palliative Care for Patients with Metastatic Non–Small-Cell Lung Cancer New England Journal of Medicine, 363:8, 8-19-2010, p733-742.

18

Hospice Care
by Ella Bittel, Holistic Veterinarian

How does hospice care for dogs compare to hospice for people?

How do I find someone to assist me with hospice for my dog?

"Heart dog" is not a term found in the dictionary, at least not yet. Anyone whose heart was ever inhabited by a dog companion, inevitably expanding his or her ability to love, will understand what I mean when I speak of Momo as my "heart dog." My many adventures with Momo could easily fill a book. Yet her greatest gift to me was defined 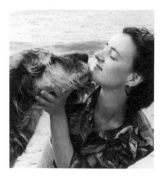 by the last chapter of her life. She passed as she had lived, following her own inner rhythm even as it slowed and ceased.

One of the reasons I became a veterinarian was to have the ability to kindly end an animal's life via euthanasia. It was reassuring to me to have the legal authority and knowledge to end otherwise unrelievable suffering. Yet when it came to Momo's last days, euthanasia didn't seem the right option.

We were together through 17 years of life's challenges, and I could read Momo about as well as she could me. At the end of her life, I was completely open to giving her what so frequently is termed the gift of euthanasia, but it turned out that euthanasia was not what she wanted.

Living day-by-day, moment-by-moment, she left it up to me to figure out what else to do.

I struggled with this, riding an emotional roller coaster between wondering if she would recover once more, as she had always done before, or if she would reach a point where she would prefer help out of her declining body with the use of drugs. Unplanned, yet in my presence, she passed in her own time. While at peace with her passing, I was left with a silent question in my mind that I could not quite put my finger on.

One day something clicked, and in an instant I realized what had felt unresolved for me. Nothing I had ever learned in veterinary school or afterward had prepared me to care for a dying being without the use of euthanasia. I knew how to fight for a life, and I knew how to take it, but I had not learned to embrace the process of supporting life even as it comes to a close. It seemed a grandiose absurdity not to have noticed that I was a one-trick pony when it came to the last season of an animal's life.

I also knew that I was far from an exception. If an animal's condition is considered terminal, veterinarians are taught as students to take control over the time of death. I certainly had witnessed enough occasions when everyone was grateful for the availability of euthanasia. But what about the idea of lovingly caring for the dying and keeping them comfortable until they leave on their own terms? Isn't that something every veterinary student ought to learn about, too?

Having deeply engaged in therapy modalities outside the norm throughout my career, I figured there must be some literature on how to care for an animal through the end of its life that I had simply not come across yet. I figured wrong. It took my own experiences with the dying to fill my toolbox, and then I began to offer the education to others that I hadn't found myself. It was not until a human hospice worker took one of my weekend seminars that I realized I was re-inventing the wheel. These concepts had been initiated half a century ago in human care and had gained momentum ever since: with hospice.

What Is Hospice?

Modern human hospice arose from the fact that the medical field had largely failed to serve the multifaceted needs of dying patients and their loved ones. Doctors and nurses are trained to work toward a cure, or at least partial recovery, in all cases, but eventually such outcomes are no longer a possibility with the terminally ill. When modern human hospice began, it came as a great blessing to this special group of patients and their families.

Hospice is a team-directed approach providing the highest level of physical, emotional and spiritual care possible to the patient and family throughout the end-of-life process. It recognizes *dying*, rather than as a failed medical event, as a natural part of the cycle of life, a process that needn't be feared or avoided. The focus is on "intensive caring," instead of "intensive care," and involves maintaining maximum comfort and quality of life without prolonging or hastening death.

Hospice helps patients, family and friends make the best of a very precious, though challenging time—a time that will remain with them as a meaningful, life long memory.

Tasks of the Hospice Team

Those who have had experience with hospice commonly say of the team, "They were angels. We could not have done it without them." Hospice can be indispensable, involving a multitude of helpful services.

With human hospice, the patient receives home visits by nurses specifically trained to provide symptom control, and the care-giving family has access to support 24/7. If symptom control becomes more challenging and the home setting won't allow for more complicated treatment, the patient may be brought into a palliative care unit with 24/7 nursing assistance. Often, the patient returns to his or her residence within a few days, with the new treatment approach in place. Even if the patient is admitted to a hospital for symptom control, the hospice team continues to provide services.

Hospice offers the entire family grief and spiritual support, as desired, and social workers help family members find the best solutions for their daily challenges, including logistical and financial issues. Respite care is available to give the family caregiver a chance to get much needed time to rest or tend to other important tasks. House aides help with light housework, volunteers may provide transportation to doctor visits, run errands or lend an open and compassionate ear, and stay at the bedside of the actively dying patient.

The needs of family members interested in hospicing their dogs are remarkably similar when their four-legged companions are dying. Some individuals and veterinary practices have taken great steps to offer end-of-life care to animals, yet services truly comparable to the ones widely available to humans are still largely to be invented. Just as medical doctors must be specifically educated to understand the distinctly different needs of the dying over those who are ill but not close to dying, veterinarians need training to learn how to properly provide hospice care, and experience to help caregivers understand the changes unfolding in their dying animal. Such veterinarians are currently still a minority.

For now, many of those wishing to deliver hospice-like treatment to their companion dog are still left mostly to their own devices to cobble together the services they need. If you find yourself in that situation, the best options to preparing are to:

- Educate yourself on animal hospice or also through human hospice resources, by volunteering, studying reputable online and printed publications, attending conferences.

- Find a veterinarian who will support your wish to, if feasible, allow your dog to die in its own time, and who will agree to offer the animal at home as much comfort and pain control as may be necessary,

- Discuss your plans well ahead with those that live together with you and your dog to get a feel for what their perspectives are.

- Find out who among the local pet sitters and your family members, friends and neighbors might be able and willing to watch your dog while you take a shower or rest, or simply support you with specific daily tasks (meals, shopping, picking up kids from school, walking your other dog/s, etc.).

- Locate an animal hospice helpline to connect with as needed.

Is Your Veterinarian Supportive of True Animal Hospice?

Giving hospice is a calling, yet it's not everyone's calling. Like individuals in any group of animal lovers, veterinarians too differ in what they feel is best for a dog. What they have been trained to do, as well as their own personal perspective on dying, influence what services they are comfortable offering. If you feel drawn to seek out hospice for your animal, have a conversation with your veterinarian about this as soon as you can.

It's always a good idea to be prepared, and even if your dog is still a puppy, it is not too early to determine if your current veterinarian will be supportive of your wishes through all of your dog's life stages.

Be specific about what you are looking for. Some veterinarians may call their services "hospice," even though they have a nearly 100 percent euthanasia rate among their "hospice" patients. If your dog experiences a health crisis such as a sudden occurrence or increase of already existing pain or breathing difficulties under hospice care, you will want a veterinarian willing to meet it with timely changes in treatment plan. For complications anticipated to arise in the future, preventative care measures are to be put in place. The veterinarian is the one to ensure that you as the caregiver get equipped with tools, in form of a "comfort kit," to meet such challenge should it occur when veterinary intervention is not in immediate reach.

A comfort kit contains fast acting strong painkillers and anti-anxiety medication in either a sublingual form or as injectables, and other drugs that can alleviate symptoms that may be anticipated if the animal's specific condition worsens. Those familiar with complementary treatment options such as homeopathy or herbs, will include such remedies and formulas for symptom control with the kit in addition to the conventional drugs.

Whether hospice is listed among the services or not, you can set up a preliminary consultation and ask your veterinarian these questions:

- Do you have personal experience caring for an animal until it passes peacefully on its own? If yes, can you tell me a little bit about that experience?

- What is your experience in guiding clients through their animal's dying process? Will you offer information about the dying process and how to care for an animal that is going through it?

- Approximately what percentage of your hospice clients are able to care for their dogs through the end of their animals' lives? Have there been undesirable outcomes? If yes, what was the cause and how could a situation like this be avoided in the future?

- Does your practice offer phone advice 24/7?

- Do you offer house visits or collaborate with other veterinarians and/or veterinary technicians to cover 24/7 in-home medical care and/or in-home euthanasia? (Note: Euthanasias generally have to be performed by a veterinarian.)

- Do you hold the necessary license permitting you to dispense controlled substances such as morphine? If yes, would you be willing to equip me with a small amount of strong, fast acting, injectable pain medications (including opiates) as one part of a comfort kit, so that I can address an acute pain crisis in my dog, should veterinary care be unavailable in a timely manner?

- Can you provide contacts of hospice clients you worked with who were successful in assisting their animals all the way to their own deaths? (While veterinarians have to protect private information, they can ask those owners for permission; typically, those who have been through such experience are very open to sharing their thoughts with those contemplating a similar endeavor.)

  - Does your practice offer integrative care? Integrative care entails both conventional (such as drugs) and complementary (such as acupuncture, homeopathy or herbal) treatment options. If the veterinary practice does not offer integrative care, ask if the veterinarian is open to work in conjunction with another vet who offers those aspects not covered.

If you find that your veterinarian, for whatever reason, is not the one to help you care for your animal in a hospice manner, ask if he or she can refer you to someone who can. Invest into paying to meet a house call veterinarian if available in your area, to engage in an end-of-life care conversation and learn about his or her responses to the above set of questions.

What Does the Dying Process Entail?

What happens during the dying process can look quite different among individuals, but it's important to note that while some terminal illnesses can involve pain, dying is not a painful process by nature. If we are not familiar with what happens at this time, however, the changes a patient goes through can easily be misinterpreted as suffering.

Below are some of the most common symptoms. It is important to note that the final physical decline in a dog may happen over a period of days, few weeks or months, but the following discussion is meant to be understood in the context of the active dying process, which generally takes place over the last few days or even just hours of life.

Mobility

It is understood that in many cases a dying patient at a certain stage can no longer rise. All throughout hospice the bedding needs to be comfortable and smooth. Using high quality foam mattresses avoids undesired clumping as so common with synthetic dog bed fillings. Having incontinence pads under both the hind and front end of the dog, in combination with use of unscented baby wipes, make for easy clean up as needed while keeping the patient as undisturbed as possible. As long as not imminently dying, the dog gets gently turned every three to four hours, though additional re-positioning will be offered if needed.

Eating

During your dog's mid-life and also throughout much of its senior years, you rightfully would be concerned if he stopped eating, particularly if the dog always had a hearty appetite. If you have cared for a dying friend or family member, chances are you have witnessed your loved one's appetite dwindle until it ceased completely, though not necessarily in linear procession. Naturally, this is usually accompanied with considerable loss of body weight.

This is also common among dogs that are close to the end of their lives. It is important to not mistake this loss of appetite for the same symptom caused by a treatable reason, or overlook it possibly being due to side effects of medications not uncommon with use of, for example, non-steroidal anti-inflammatory drugs (NSAIDS) or antibiotics. For a period of time at the beginning of hospice, a dog may still accept food customized to his change in appetite, by using different ingredients, changing the texture or temperature of the food, and offering it by hand, from a lifted bowl or off a spoon. A dog may also skip eating a meal for a day or two, and then accept something again. This is a time when creativity and having another dog to take care of leftovers go a long way. But at some point it is common for a dying individual to stop eating entirely.

While it may make you uncomfortable to witness a loved one moving one step closer toward death, it is important you are internally prepared for recognizing and accepting loss of appetite inside the active dying process. If you don't understand that the dying simply no longer feel hungry once their body can no longer properly process and benefit from food, you might mistake this for starving and start force feeding or think you have to euthanize your dog.

It is important to realize that force feeding the dying causes them discomfort, and can lead to nausea, vomiting, bloating, diarrhea, even breathing difficulties.

You can offer a variety of foods intermittently in case your dog changes its mind and wants to take some voluntarily, just make sure to remove them from the room if declined, as even just the scents can trigger nausea. In the very end, "eating right" for the dying often means "eating nothing."

Drinking and Hydration

Loss of thirst in actively dying humans and animals including dogs is very common. At this time, giving fluids to the patient who will not take them voluntarily becomes a life-prolonging measure, it may hinder a smooth transition. During most of life, dehydration is frequently associated with discomfort which can be relieved by fluids. Hydration is used also in hospice, but only if and for as long as it improves comfort levels. Whether human or animal, forcing hydration when the patient's body can no longer properly absorb fluids can lead to edemas, nausea, vomiting and difficulty breathing. With increasing dehydration, medications may need to be adjusted. If the mouth gets dry, it can be moistened with the help of a wet cotton swab if that appears to add to the dog's comfort.

> *Lack of thirst commonly occurs some time after the lack of interest in food may occur, indicating your loved one is yet one step closer to the final goodbye.*

Unless interest in drinking recurs in your dog, in the absence of forced hydration, the hours are counted, and this can be an utmost precious time to spend together and express our love once more.

Interaction

We have come to expect our dogs to respond to us when calling their names, and to give us visible signals that they are happy to see us, such as turning their heads toward us, perking their ears and wagging their tails. These gestures give us joy and let us know our dogs are well. But if you have spent time at the bedside of a dying human loved one, you may have noticed that they tend to rest and sleep a lot. Even when awake, their focus may shift between being present to us and gazing at things invisible to our eyes.

Just as people, it then is common for dogs to remain in a resting position. There may come a time when they do this with their eyes remaining at least partially open, it then is best to keep light levels dim. We know from humans that at this point blankets can feel very heavy, so if at all needed for your dog, use only very light and loose covers.

Besides continuing to provide quietly and gently for hygiene as needed, ensure that noise levels are kept to a minimum, for example by turning the ringer of the phone down, muffling the door bell, and having noisy younger dog companions temporarily stay with a friend. While many of us have been exposed to the romantic notion of "dying in the arms of our beloved," it turns out that some of the dying prefer to no longer be touched though they may not be able to express that by moving away anymore, so remain aware of that possibility.

These are some of the common occurrences during the dying process. Quality-of-life scales as currently used in veterinary medicine to determine when to euthanize, list normal signs of dying as described above among the reasons to euthanize, and are therefore not applicable in animal hospice. If experienced in hospice, your veterinarian can explain additional typical symptoms when preparing you to care for your dog during its transition, else you can find this information by getting in touch with an animal hospice helpline.

Can You Do It? Find Out!

"Start by doing what's necessary, then do what's possible,
and suddenly you are doing the impossible."
– Saint Francis of Assisi

Especially when new to hospice, you can't really know how you will hold up to the emotional, physical and other challenges of giving this special care until you are doing it. Some suggest dog owners ponder ahead of time what physical and mental changes in their animal they would be willing to deal with and where they would draw the line. This is not helpful to do in preparation for giving hospice, as it would limit yourself to who you are in that moment, freezing your capacity to expand.

I have found myself completely underestimating people's capacity to manage major care challenges. Some avoid reading a book that entails the death of an animal yet grow to any challenge when it comes to their own animal's declining health. Looking back to their animal's time of passing, many caregivers note that they could not have anticipated being able to do what they did.

> *A common comment of those successful in supporting an animal all the way through its time of passing is, "It was the hardest thing I have ever done, and I would do it again in a heartbeat."*

If you stay in the moment and deal with what is at hand, you will find out what you can and cannot do at that moment in time. Remember: what you are able to do during hospice often is influenced by the support available to you. This is one of the reasons why it is so critical to prepare ahead of time. Educate yourself and locate your resources. Find out who could be players on your support team before you need that support.

Keeping All Options Open

You cannot ever completely predict what awaits you as you accompany your dog during its last days of life. Even if your heart and mind are set to allow your animal to go in its own time, it is important to have a Plan B in place and accessible 24/7, and to remain open to choose it. In those exceptions where a dog's comfort cannot be sufficiently managed, hospice care may still have to be concluded by euthanasia. Not everyone who hopes to care for a dog until it can peacefully pass on its own will find they are able to do so. Time, as well as physical, emotional and financial limitations may become obstacles, leading a caregiver to consider euthanasia. This can trigger feelings of guilt, as well as a sense of failure. If that happens, remember this:

Whether you allow an animal to die in its own time by providing hospice or choose euthanasia, you base your decision on what you find yourself able to provide and perceive is best for your beloved animal. It is important to have compassion for yourself at all times. Questions of life and death are too big to fit into black and white categories.

If you are in emotional distress over watching your dog's health deteriorate and are considering euthanasia for its benefit, it is of essence to keep these two questions distinct:

- Is your dog in discomfort or suffering?
- Does your dog still want to live?

Even if the answer is "yes" to the first question, the answer to the second one may well be "no." Just as common in humans, a dog too may want to live, in spite of suffering. It is wise to avoid making final decisions when you have any doubts or are under great distress. Instead, allow yourself and your family time to come to terms with the situation, even if that means asking the veterinarian for further pain control or other comfort measures instead of immediately following a euthanasia suggestion. With a clear head and a quiet mind, you can best perceive your dog's wishes and perhaps even find ways to solve care challenges when everyone else says it's impossible.

No matter what your decision, you, as the loving caregiver of your dog, deserve to be fully supported and respected. At this most tender time, when you are losing the physical presence of your beloved animal, the last thing you need is someone judging you for the path you choose and influencing you to do something you may feel guilty about later.

Hospice as a Gift also to the Caregiver

Those considering giving hospice can be assured that it can be a remarkable journey. This brief discussion cannot capture the preciousness, so palpable in their presence, of a dying animal's remaining hours and days. When it came to Momo, I was willing to give her the gift of euthanasia, but she instead gave me the gift of engaging with that part of our life called *dying*, opening my eyes to a whole new world of living and caring. Laura G. from Portland, OR, a caregiver, who took my seminar and subsequently chose to give hospice to her dear dog Kaya when he was diagnosed with advanced cancer, articulated this eloquently:

Kaya gave me so many gifts; unconditional love, of course, was the greatest among them. And his final one, allowing me to share his natural passing ... we were given the grace needed in those hours, to experience one of the greatest mysteries in life, the ending. If you have the good fortune that your dear companion animal does not die by an accident, that there is not unbearable pain, that you can be present ... it is an amazing gift. A chance to peek into that portal, where we are going. A sacred transition. You will be forged stronger, deeper, more accepting than you ever imagined. And yes, you will be more ready, for next time, whose ever time it will be.

Ella Bittel, born in Germany followed her childhood desire to help animals by becoming a veterinarian. Now living and working in Arizona and California, Ella has specialized in holistic modalities for over 25 years, among them veterinary acupuncture and chiropractic, cranio-sacral work, homeopathy and TTOUCH. When Momo, Ella's dog companion of 17 years, reached the end of her life, it became clear to Ella that none of her expansive veterinary training had included education on how to support an animal throughout its own dying process. Her experiences with caring for Momo all the way to her self–determined passing—and Ella's deep sense that, just like birth, the dying process can be of inherent value and an important part of an individual's journey—led her to engage in animal hospice. She created much needed educational resources including online classes for anyone interested in options in end-of life care for animal companions, for more info go to www.spiritsintransition.org. Ella's vision is that a network of support will be developed on a national and worldwide scale for those choosing hospice care for a terminally ill animal family member. Besides nationwide presentations of her weekend seminar "Spirits in Transition," Ella Bittel has been a speaker on the topic of animal hospice at various professional conferences, including the

2010 AVMA convention and the First and Second International Symposium for Veterinary Hospice Care at UC Davis.

1050 S. Page Springs Rd., Suite B
Cornville, AZ 86325
(928) 634-2707
www.SpiritsInTransition.org
SpiritsInTransition@verizon.net

My Favorite Resources:

Bright Haven Healing Arts Center for Animals
  www.BrightHaven.org

The Nikki Hospice Foundation for Pets
  www.PetHospice.org

American Holistic Veterinary Medical Assn.
  www.AHVMA.org

Pet Loss Help
  www.PetLossHelp.org

ASPCA Phone Pet Loss Support
  ph. (877) 474-3310

The Senior Dog Project
  www.SRDogs.com

Wheelchairs for Dogs
  www.Doggon.com

Products for Dogs with Special Needs
  www.HandicappedPets.com

Therapeutic and Rehabilitative Products
www.DogLeggs.com

Canine Cancer and more
  www.LandOfPureold.com

Tellington-TTouch
  www.TTouch.com

19

Pet Home Euthanasia
with Dr. Michelle Morrison (Dr. MiMi)

Will I have time to say good-bye the way I want to?

Should I be present during the euthanasia?

"I am grateful for this life, everyday."
– Dr. MiMi

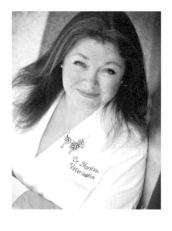

The service of pet home euthanasia is a relatively new offering. Most people do not know it is available across the country. While the idea is unknown to many, the concept is quite simple: Rather than take your pet to the family veterinarian's office for his last moments, a veterinarian comes to your home for the service. My experience is that it is a much more desirable alternative way to approach your animal's transition.

When my clients ask me how I can offer euthanasia as a service, I say "I get to be around love, everyday." Putting dogs "to sleep" is emotionally hard on veterinarians and performing euthanasia takes strength on the part of any veterinarian. Don't be surprised if we shed a tear with you. Yet this is nothing compared to the courage and fortitude that my clients and patients must endure to get through the eminent separation from one another, the last loving moment when they have to say good-bye for the very final time. Being sensitive to the struggles they are facing, I go to them with reverence. I am grateful and honored to be the one chosen at that time for each person and their pet.

As a veterinarian who practices holistic medicine, I never give up on the hope of life. But that is not the position I am in when an owner calls me for euthanasia. At that point, the focus is on an animal that is clearly and irreversibly declining. An animal chaplain I know said she believes that owners pick up the phone and call me because their pet is communicating their readiness to pass over or transition. A myriad of questions come forth including: "How do I know when it is the right time?" or "What do I say to my children?"

Feelings of guilt, wondering if they waited too long or not long enough are common.

As a traditional veterinarian with a holistic, alternative philosophy, I begin by discussing the medical conditions, the prognosis or outcome of those medical conditions and then help my clients gauge the severity of their pet's condition. Together, we total up the problems and see if the moment is close. I embellish the medical condition with spiritual, social and psychological considerations to make each situation concentrate on a more "whole" life approach. My potential clients—friends on the other end of the telephone—are grateful at the end of our initial conversation. I have helped them clearly understand where they are at this point of the decision. Every situation is true and correct for them alone—it may not be true for the next person.

To help someone with the struggle of making the decision, I may recommend that additional medical advice from the family veterinarian is obtained. Their veterinarian is most familiar with their dog's situation and may have performed a recent examination supporting that the owner's intuition is correct and it is the right time for euthanasia.

> *I urge my clients to trust their own instincts and their own hearts. They are the designated guardians for their pets, and no one on this planet could take better care of their pets.*

This makes them the final and best judge, not me. I simply provide the details of the process involved with in-home euthanasia.

Euthanasia done in your home provides a more peaceful and relaxing environment for you and your pet. It allows you to take the time you and your family need for acceptance and healing. Time for saying good-bye in the home usually takes around one hour (or a little longer), from beginning to end. In addition to being in a comfortable and familiar setting, your pet will appreciate not having to take a bumpy car ride that jostles their joints and causes them pain. They get to transition at home, where they feel safe.

Every in-home euthanasia veterinarian is special in their own way. He or she will bring personality, experience and excellence to the appointment and concentrate on what is best for the client. I believe you are meant to feel a connection with a particular veterinarian when you speak with them or read their website and you choose them with your heart. I always say, "You are meant to find the one right for you." This means that no service will be the same or be exactly as I would perform my service. Each will vary in the time spent with you.

From the choice of medications that affect the time from the sedation process to the euthanasia process and whether or not a catheter is used will be determined. An I.V. catheter may be avoided and is not always necessary unless indicated by the choice of medication. You can trust that your in-home euthanasia veterinarian will be very experienced handling the medications and the needs and medical condition of your pet.

The following is a detailed look at my specific in-home care euthanasia. I offer my clients the knowledge gained from 15 years of experience, giving them psychological support from my grief and loss training enhanced with a holistic twist.

Making the Appointment

Beginning with the first call to discuss making an appointment, I make sure to cover all of the details with them. Every family's needs are different. First, each person must search his or her own heart and decide if they want to be present for the euthanasia. I have found that some people will not attend—not because of a lack of love, but just the opposite. They love their dogs so deeply, it breaks their heart to be present and watch what they imagine to be an unpleasant event (which it is not). While everyone is given the freedom to do what they feel is most appropriate, the majority stay. Either choice is fine with me.

Parents are often surprised when I recommend that they do not hide the euthanasia from their children and, instead, ask them what their heart is telling them to do. Surprisingly, to all, many are comfortable and wish to stay. If they do, the event can create a better family bond and understanding of death, as well as help with acceptance.

Don't be surprised when children choose to take part in all aspects of the euthanasia process. They ask good questions, help lift their pet, take pictures at the beautiful last look and some even lay with them the entire time.

Another issue I cover at this time is what sort of setting the client prefers for the euthanasia. I advise them to pick a setting where the family, as well as other family pets, will feel welcome and comfortable; to think about any special requests they may have for their pet's end-of-life transition; and to include music, flowers, favorite toys near their dog and prayers. They might even deliver a eulogy. I offer to leave the room to allow total privacy for all.

In the initial phone call, I also discuss bringing a technician to the home to help lift a heavy dog. The client may feel physically (and emotionally) able to lift their dog, preferring a more intimate setting with less people (strangers) in their home. We also go over the fees for euthanasia, cremation or burial options, choice of individualized urns and if they want a memorable paw print in a photo frame.

The In-home Appointment

When I come for the in-home appointment, I am often greeted at the door by other family pets. I will acknowledge those happy pets by offering them a treat after they sit politely. This helps them settle down and accept me as a person who understands their needs; they regard me as a friend from this moment on. Sometimes the Beloved Pet greets me, too (I don't make them sit). At other times, the Beloved Pet may bark or communicate with me from a lying down position or just wag his tail. I approach him on my knees and offer my hand, which holds a delicious, dehydrated, raw food treat. Generally, even dogs that have not eaten in days will take my gift. If not, they still appreciate the offer and regard me as a friend. I introduce myself to the family with hugs of support, and we all surround the Beloved Pet on the floor. I then give a description of what will happen along the way and what they will witness.

The appointment begins with filling out the permission/authorization form, which includes the name they want on the urn (if they want the cremains/ashes returned). I also review the client's preferences for cremation after-care choices. "Simple cremation" does not include the return of cremains. The "individual cremation" service cremates more than one pet at one time. Up to three will be cremated together, but they are expertly kept separate and only the Beloved Pet's cremains are returned in the urn. (I've found this is the most popular choice.) A "private cremation" is chosen by those who want to have their pet cremated solely. The cremation company I use even has an option which allows the owners to be present at the time to watch the cremation. Very few choose this option, yet some owners appreciate this for the emotional peace. I also offer a clay paw-print in a photo frame, made by my technician, as an elegant memorial to their Beloved Pet.

A history is gathered of how the owners arrived at their decision with the medical conditions leading up to this moment. I also perform a brief and gentle examination of their pet. Cardiovascular and respiratory systems are assessed to determine the type and amount of sedation necessary. Out of respect for the pet's last moments, and to avoid any painful spots which may irritate the pet during the euthanasia, I will palpate the abdomen and examine masses or musculoskeletal problems after the pet has passed. A post-euthanasia examination is performed because some clients have not seen their family veterinarian before the decision to euthanize. They may be unaware that their pet has, for example, evidence of cancer. When I make them aware of the severity of anything I note, the owners are grateful and feel confirmation of their decision.

Sedation

Before the sedation, I advise my clients to take time to express loving words; they might say a prayer or convey love and appreciation for all their pet has meant to them in their lives, whispering sweet words and letting the pet know it is okay to pass over.

Then, I will ask the Beloved Pet to say good-bye to each family member present. This is the most beautiful thing I have ever witnessed, as each pet will look up into the eyes of his people and communicate, in his own special way, a sense of good-bye. Words cannot describe this connection, this communion. I only know that my clients feel peace at a level unimaginable, because of this last loving moment that aids them in the acceptance of this phase of life. I will then ask the dog's permission to allow me to help him pass over. Many times, pets will lay their heads down and even close their eyes, telling the family and me that they are ready. Some actually look happy. Most have a look of acceptance and understanding and they are okay to go. As I begin, none look afraid.

It is my objective that your pet should never experience any pain, discomfort or fear throughout the euthanasia process. Therefore, I provide the pet a sedative. It is the first of two injections I will give. The sedation and time I allow will put them into a peaceful, comforting and deep sleep which involves body twitching and snoring. The sedation type and amount will be based on the pet's physical condition. I explain any complications we may see from the sedation or final anesthesia based on their pet's condition.

Owners relax as they understand that all is under control and they are not to worry. I proceed with the sedation process only after all their questions have been answered. Animals feel very relaxed and free of pain, and their owners are more comfortable seeing them in this state. Many owners state, "I have not seen them this comfortable for months..." For dogs, this sedation takes full effect in approximately 20 minutes. My choice of sedation for this painless injection, placed right under the skin like a vaccine, is butorphanol (effects like morphine) and acepromazine (given to dogs before a plane flight or for thunderstorm anxiety).

Once the pet is sedated with the initial shot, we wait 20 minutes. The Beloved Pet is stroked and petted as we speak softly to him. At this time, we have a final celebration of life while he is still with us in a peaceful state. Some clients show me pictures of when the dog was in his prime or during a funny moment. Others tell happy stories or remain silent; whatever the family desires.

Euthanasia

After 20 minutes, I assess the pet and inquire if my clients are ready. I offer to give them some more private time with their pet. Once my clients feel they are ready, I will proceed with putting their beloved pet to final rest. A second injection (sodium pentobarbital, a general anesthetic drug used for pets) is given into a vein which courses through the heart and affects the brain. The brain responds immediately and the pet is unconscious and unaware. It takes effect in only a few moments (around seven seconds) and the breathing slows and heart stops. I will listen to the pet's heart and let everyone know when the pet has passed. Out of respect to some owners, I allow anyone to feel free to confirm that the heart has stopped by feeling near the elbow or I will let them auscult with my stethoscope. Most people decline and trust me.

Afterward is what I call "family time." I encourage family members to take time to hold their pet or lay against him—whatever is needed for each individual and the family as a whole. There is no need to hurry. I have spent up to four hours at a client's home answering questions, going over medical conditions, consulting with their veterinarians and giving all family members as much time as they need.

Next, it is time for the pet members of the family. If clients have other dogs or animals in the home, it often helps these pets' understanding to allow them to see and acknowledge their friend's passing. And yes, this is where I receive the most skepticism. But clients who allow their pets to take this time are always surprised and happy that they've listened to my suggestion to do so. There is a special way of assuring that your other pets gain a healthy acceptance of their friend's transition. This begins with an understanding of what I call "the spirit circle" that surrounds your deceased pet. The spirit circle cannot be seen by us, but I believe it is felt, or smelled, by your pets. It is best to take one pet at a time up to the nose area of your deceased pet. By sniffing this area, pets usually understand that their friend has passed.

I then ask the owner to gently push each pet, one more time, toward the nose. If that pet stiffens and refuses to be pushed closer toward their friend, or if they turn their head or look away, they know their friend has passed. They exhibit this behavior out of respect to the spirit circle and they will not cross it, no matter how hard you push them. Before the pets walk away, I instruct the clients to embrace them, look them directly in the eyes and say, "I am sorry." This is a magical phrase that lets the surviving pets know you understand that their friend has passed. The pets will usually lick your face. I cannot explain any of this. I only know what I see every day. It is one of the sweetest moments I have had the privilege to observe. Surviving family pets have amazing acceptance and will wag their tails and act happier after we perform this little ceremony for them. They understand and they are okay.

Beautiful, Last Look

When everyone in the family feels comfortable letting their pet leave the home, I ask if anyone desires to help me carry their dog to my vehicle (or I enlist the help of my technician). Most clients want to be involved; afterward, I ask them to go back into the home for a few minutes as I wish to surprise them.

In just a few minutes, I place their pet in billowing, soft, white fluffy blankets. The Beloved Pet's head is laid to rest on a white satin pillow with a feather boa draped around his body. Colorful teddy bears are added as final decorations. I ask the owners if their pet has a special stuffed animal or ball which they would want to place between his paws as a symbol of love. Some clients have chosen flowers from the garden, tennis balls, slippers or a special toy.

They exclaim when they see this and start to cry a little more, then smiles spread across their faces. This is the time that they really hug me and let me know how much they appreciate the respect I have given their pet. Almost everyone takes a photo, capturing the sweet beauty of their pet in a cozy, fresh setting. I assure them it is healthy to take all the photos they want.

After the euthanasia, I advise all owners to take special care of themselves in the days to follow. They have been through a great deal of stress and this takes a toll on their bodies, especially their adrenal glands (I recommend hot bubble baths with candles or a soak in the jacuzzi). I wish them love and blessings and let them know I am here for them at any time. I tell them I have a list of supportive experts who are ready for a call from them, if needed, and I recommend they watch the Rainbow Bridge video on my website *www.PetHomeEuthanasia.com*, when they are ready. Final hugs are given and I depart.

When Hospice Is the Alternative

In addition to in-home euthanasia, I also provide in-home hospice. Some people (and pets) decide that it is just not the right time. For example, I was once called to the home of Gizmo. When I arrived, the dog ran behind her owner to hide from me. Gizmo was not ready to leave on that day. Another dog, a Chihuahua, growled at me and ran to eat her food, as if to say, "See, I'm eating, I am fine!" In both of these instances, their scheduled euthanasia was postponed.

Another famous patient of mine involved a Rocko the Rottweiler with Osteosarcoma. His owners were diligent in trying to save his life. Rocko underwent radiation therapy and after three weeks from the completion of treatment, we were to begin my other cancer supplements for support (very important not to interfere with the radiation process). He, unfortunately, fractured his leg at the site of the cancer.

The owners did not want to amputate his leg or give up and have him euthanized because he was happy, healthy and strong due to the excellent nutritional support and supplements I had prescribed. They elected to try everything, so we began using the Magnafix PEMF unit and his bone fracture hardened and continued laying down more new bone for months that could be seen on radiographs. Rocko survived for many months and had an excellent quality of life until his last day.

Not everyone believes in euthanasia. I didn't, but I have changed my beliefs. I see my clients' acceptance and I hope that as more people experience the love and peacefulness of an in-home pet euthanasia, they will learn to accept death as a natural process that can be honored in a positive way. More importantly, I thank my clients who choose me to be present with them. It is an honor.

Dr. Michelle Morrison is a 15-year licensed veterinarian working in Phoenix, Arizona for over 11 years and is known as Dr. Mimi. She attended Michigan State University undergraduate in pre-vet. She received her Doctor of Veterinary Medicine (DVM) at the University of Tennessee in 1995. Dr. Morrison now owns and operates a mobile veterinary practice in Scottsdale.

She is a traditional, western medicine veterinarian with a broader scope of healing modalities with an alternative slant to help animals prolong and enhance their quality of life. One aspect of her practice includes the honor of being present with pets and their owners and performing beautiful, home pet euthanasias. She received the 2011 Outstanding Practice Award in Veterinary Medicine for her Pet Home Euthanasia service. Other practices used in conjunction include but are not limited to: Certified Veterinary Chiropractitioner (CVCP), Cold Laser (Erchonia), Homotoxicology which includes BioPuncture (homepathy directed into affected areas), herbal medicine (Chinese, Western and Ayruvedic), Bicom Machine, Reiki, Applied Kinesiology, along with wide selection of her favorite supplements to maintain optimum health or stimulate the immune system (for cancer patients).

Dr. Morrison utilizes a new machine and methodology, the Magnafix (PEMF) technology, which uses a new wave form that has never been used before and has been accelerating healing times in disc disease, fractures, soft tissue leg injuries (ACL), shortening infection time, lengthening some cancer patients lifespan and boosting the immune system response. You can learn more about her experiences and the continuing myriad of disease conditions of the Magnafix unit and other combination modalities at www.TheHolisticVet.net.

Pet Home Euthanasia
11445 E. Via Linda Avenue, Suite 2233
Scottsdale, Arizona 85259
623-680-9200
DrMimi@PetHomeEuthanasia.com

My Favorite Resources:

American Holistic Veterinary Medical Association
www.ahvma.com

In Home Pet Euthanasia Directory - 50 states
www.InHomePetEuthanasia.com

Rainbow Bridge Movie by Terry Pike and Kerry Muzzey
www.RainbowBridge.com

Memorializing your dog-Post on-line memorials
www.ILovedMyPet.com

Clay Paws
www.ClayPaws.com
800-827-6985

Pet Urns
www.4GoodWorks.com
www.CheersPottery.com

Internat. Assoc. for Animal Hospice and Palliative Care
www.iaahpc.org
www.AngelAnimals.com

Plaques
www.ReflectionsInTime.net

Memorial Pet Resources
www.iaahpc.org
www.In-Memory-of-pets.com
www.MyCherishedPet.com
www.Paws2Heaven.com
www.Perpetualpet.net
www.CelebrativeArt.com

Memory Markers
www.BrandNewPetMarkers.com

International Association of Pet Cemeteries
518-594-3000

Grief Counselors
www.aplb.org.
www.DeltaSociety.org
www.Pet-Loss.net

Self Healing Expressions – Grief Resources and Books
www.SelfHealingExpressions.com

Visit the Prayers, Healing & Support Community
www.BestFriends.org

Animal Communicator
www.Listen2Animals.com

Eric's Hope Book– Fictional story based upon a true story
by Andrea Chilcote
www.EriksHope.com

20

Ceremony Ideas for Animals by Frances Fitzgerald Cleveland, EOS, HP

How can a ceremony help with grief?

Can you give me some ideas on how to create my own ceremony?

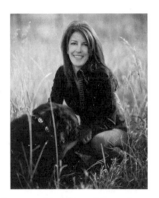

One fall, my 28-year-old Morgan horse Pete became very sick. He was in a great deal of pain, very weak and not able to stand. We tried for 24 hours to help him get through this strange illness. I spent the night in Pete's stall talking and singing to him. He quietly laid there listening and sighing every now and then. As the sun started to rise and light illuminated his stall, I whispered to him, "Hey Pete, the sun is rising. It's going to be a beautiful day. How about you getting up too?" Pete just stared at me with a beautiful calmness, and in my heart I knew he was ready to go. My husband John also noticed how peaceful Pete was and said, "That is the quietest I have seen him in the past 24 hours."

The vet arrived and began explaining the invasive technique she was going to perform to get Pete up on all fours and into a harness. Holding back the tears, I said, "But look how quiet and peaceful he is." She then gently said to me, "You only have one other option." John and I knew intuitively that Pete's tranquility signaled that he was ready to go, even though we were not. Thinking back to my recent trip to Belize where I had learned about spiritual and healing ceremonies with plants, I realized we needed our own ceremony or ritual to aid Pete and ourselves in his passing.

After telling my vet that we needed some time to say good-bye, I went to my garden and found some plants that were still growing. One of them happened to be rosemary, a symbol of regeneration which the Greeks and Romans believed gave comfort to the living and peace to the dead. I then selected some essential oils and my copal resin for smudging.

For our goodbye ceremony, I infused a bowl of water with rosemary, hay, and essential oils of rose, myrrh and frankincense for a spiritual bath. I braided rosemary into his mane and tail and then burned the copal resin in his stall while we were saying our goodbyes. It was a beautiful and peaceful moment that I believe greatly eased Pete. This experience convinced me that ceremony and ritual have the potential to help all animals. After all, our animals are a blessing in our lives and it only makes sense to honor them in this way.

Your Ceremony

Although my first ceremony was to aid in an animal's passing, ceremonies and rituals can be performed for many other occasions as well. A ceremony can welcome a newly acquired animal into your life and help it let go of the life it left to come into yours. If you foster animals, a ceremony can be a beautiful way to say goodbye and bless them as they move into their new life. The hardest ceremony of all is, of course, saying goodbye as an animal passes on to the next realm.

When I prepare to perform a ceremony for one of my animals or for a friend's, I plan for a daylong event or, at the very least, a half day. This is a time set aside for myself, the animal and the people who are invited to participate in this special moment.

First, I choose my setting. If the weather is agreeable, I find a spot outside and place my ceremony blanket in the middle to form a circle for us all to sit around. I gather plants, tying the bundles for the plant brushings with a special ribbon and placing them in a beautiful vase (I always make a plant bundle for each person attending the ceremony).

Next, I place the plants chosen for the spiritual bath in a crystal bowl filled with water, and then set the bowl in the sun, along with a special cloth that I use for the bath. I gather my smudging materials and set them in the circle. I also place pictures and mementos of my animals that have already passed on alongside significant objects relating to the animal the ceremony is being conducted for. These items can be things such as collars, favorite toys or their favorite treats. As participants arrive, I ask them to spend a few minutes walking the yard and collecting any plants they might like to contribute to the spiritual bath.

When the bath is ready, I add two drops each of the following essential oils: frankincense, myrrh, rose and sweet marjoram; I call this my Peace Blend. Then I will place the completed bath in the center of the circle.

Once the center of the circle is complete, everyone is in attendance and our special animal has been welcomed, we begin the ceremony. I go around the circle and smudge everyone by waving a feather over the smoke so it covers the person, and during this time I am saying an opening poem or singing a song. Each participant then introduces him or herself and says something about the animal that the ceremony is being held for. I welcome the spirit of all the animals whose photos are in the center of the circle to the ceremony. Then we give the animal present a spiritual bath and a very light plant brushing, always mindful of how the animal is receiving the bath and the plant brushing and adjusting them according to their response. I quietly talk to the animal expressing my love and gratitude for them and if someone has something to add, it will be during this time.

Once this part of the ceremony is finished, everyone sits in silence with love in their hearts. This is my time to connect with the animal in a quiet state. When the silence is broken, we all stand in a circle and perform a plant brushing on each participant with them standing in the center of the circle as we gently brush them with our plant bundles and sing a song. When we have completed giving the last person their plant brushing, we smudge everyone and close the ceremony. The end of your ceremony is yours to decide. If you are having a goodbye ceremony with your animal whose time it is to pass on, you may wish for your vet to be present and say your final goodbye at the end of the ceremony, or you can wait for everyone to leave and then say your goodbyes privately.

> *It is your ceremony, and you can shape it in whatever way feels most appropriate to you and your animal.*

Unfortunately, sometimes our animals choose to leave suddenly and there is no time to prepare for a ceremony. If this is the case, you can create a quick ritual with the plants around your home, or any essential oil you may have available. Frankincense is a good one to have on hand, and I always have my Peace Blend with me. With these simple plants and oils, you can create a blessing and say your special goodbye.

With our horse Pete, we had little time to prepare and I simply did what I could at the moment. After his passing, I created a little altar in his stall on an upturned water bucket. I placed a crystal, carrots and rosemary on it and I continued to burn the copal resin in my smudge bowl every day for a week. To this day there is still a purple ribbon tied to his stall door.

In another situation with one of my animals, his passing was sudden and we were out of town. Our dog Merlin decided to pass on at our home in Colorado while we were on vacation in Rhode Island. I found two small glass bowls in the cottage we were staying in and I gave one to my husband and kept one for myself. We walked around the yard of the cottage gathering plants. We found red clover, wild rose, yellow flowers, pine needles, and purple chicory flowers to place in these two spiritual bath bowls. I then made a little altar on a table out in the sun and tended to these little bowls of love the entire week we were there.

On our last day on vacation, we poured the spiritual baths into a beautiful pitcher and walked to our favorite spot on the beach where we tearfully said our goodbyes to Merlin. We poured this spiritual bath water on our feet and onto the sand and watched the waves carry all the plants and water out to the ocean. It was one of the most beautiful and painful moments of my life, and a wonderful way to honor Merlin's spirit even though we could not be physically present. I was also grateful to know that our house-sitter at the time had the Peace Blend on hand and had given it to Merlin during this time of his passing.

If you are having a ceremony during the winter and you live in a place where the plants go dormant, you can purchase some at the flower store, or you can use plants you have dried in seasons past; I collect my marigolds, basil, rue, sage, yarrow and other plants during the growing season and dry them for use as tea or for use in ceremonies. The trees want to take part in these ceremonies, so if it resonates include them too. I always buy fresh roses for the center piece of the ceremonial circle and for the plant brushings. You can be very creative during the winter months.

All of these ceremony ideas can be performed before, during or after your animal companion has moved on. You can also perform a ceremony on the anniversary of their passing.

I have performed ceremonies for animals that have been newly adopted, had to be given away, had passed on years before, who were lost and for animals in the wild. Ceremonies are personal so feel free to create your own unique ritual to honor your animal. Much peace and love to you and your animals.

Ideas to Help You Design Your Own Personal Ceremony

Plants are a main component in all my ceremonies. They offer the healing, support, love and the peace we need, especially when we ask them to take part in our lives. Plant medicine and plant spirits have been part of daily life for centuries. I feel that in today's world, surrounded by technology and social media, it is especially important to reconnect with the plant world again. The plants are waiting for you.

Spiritual Bath

A spiritual bath is method of blending water with plants to create a beautiful way of sending healing and love to the recipient. Fill a bowl with water, add plants to this water and let sit for 15 to 30 minutes. Ideally, let the bowl sit in the sun. Use plants that have meaning to you and your animal companion. You can also just walk through your garden or flower store with the intention "which plants would like to be part of this ceremony" in your mind. Suggested plants to use are marigolds, basil, roses, rosemary, rue and any plants your animal particularly responded to. You can also add a few drops of essential oil into this spiritual bath water. Some essential oils to consider are frankincense, myrrh, rose, sweet marjoram or one of your animal's favorite essential oils.

How do you know what your animal's favorite plants or essential oils are? Notice if your animal tends to be drawn toward particular plants or smells. I had a dog who always chewed on my echinacea plants and my horse Pete loved to eat the yarrow in the garden. When I had the essential oil violet leaf on my hand, my dog Merlin would lick at it and our horse Bo loves to smell its scent and lick at my hand too.

How to use your spiritual bath: Gently massage the herbal spiritual bath water on your animal. You can use your hand or a special cloth. Only use a small amount of the water: it is a blessing, not an actual bath and you do not need to soak the animal with water. Follow your instincts when you are massaging this special water onto your animal; perhaps you may wish to apply some to yourself and the other participants in this ceremony. Sing a song, recite a poem or say a prayer during this sacred time.

Plant Brushing: Brushing is a wonderful way of using the plants to offer healing, support, love and peace to the recipient. Find plants that have special meaning to you and your animal companion. Gather a sprig of each plant and make a bundle with them; you may wish to make a plant bundle for everyone participating in your ceremony or have them make their own. As you gently brush your animal companion's body with these plants, you can say, "I have faith in all my heart of the great healing powers of … (name the plants)", sing a song, recite a poem, or just speak to the animal. Suggested plants to use are marigold, basil, rose, rosemary and rue.

Working with copal, frankincense, and myrrh resins and smudging herbs: Gather your incense burner. If you wish you may place sand in your burner, light a charcoal briquette designed for burning resin and place it on the sand (the briquette will take about 10 minutes to fully heat up. It should be a light grey color when ready to use.) When the briquette is hot, add resins and herbs at your discretion. (I prefer to have the smudge burning from the beginning to end of the ceremony.)

At the beginning and end of your ceremony, smudge all who are present. Smudging is a method of letting the smoke of the resin and herbs float over your entire body; it is a way to ground and cleanse us. Holding the smudging bowl, start at the top of the individual's head, move down to the bottom of their feet and back up again, letting the smoke gently waft over them. Lightly smudge the animal at least four times during course of the ceremony and especially at the end. If the animal is not enjoying the smudging, then just lightly smudge the surrounding area. When you are smudging, you may wish to use a feather or your hand as a wand to wave the smoke around.

Plant Suggestions to Use in Your Ceremony and their Meanings

Basil (Ocimum basilicum): A plant that is known to comfort the heart, mind and spirit.

Copal (Bursera microphylla): This resin has been used ritually by Mesoamericans for centuries. It is burned year-round in Mexican churches and is especially popular in homes during the Day of the Dead celebrations. Copal resin is traditionally burned in protection, cleansing and purification ceremonies. Large amounts of copal were burned on top of the Aztec and Mayan pyramids.

Frankincense (Boswellia carteri) and **Myrrh** (Commiphora myrrha): Since antiquity these resins have been burned to create sacred smoke that rises as a bridge between the spirits of this world and the heavens. The oil of frankincense was used in ancient Egypt to anoint the head of the dead or dying. The resins and oils are both used ceremonially to help dying animals or people move on to the next realm. Frankincense and myrrh help close the wounds of loss and rejection.

Lavender (Lavandula angustifolia): Lavender is considered the balancer of emotions. Rudolph Steiner suggests that lavender stabilizes the Physical, Etheric and Astral bodies.

Marigolds (Tagetes patula): Mesoamericans believe this is the only flower the dead can smell. Marigolds are believed to comfort the heart and the spirit.

Rose (Rosa damascena): This plant represents love and protection. In the eighth century B.C. epic poem, "The Iliad," Homer tells us how Hector's body was anointed with rose oil after his death at Achilles' hand. Rose is helpful in times of sadness, grief, disappointment and great joy.

Rosemary (Rosmarinus officinalis): The Greeks and Romans saw this plant as a symbol of regeneration; they held it to be a sacred plant. They believed this plant gave comfort to the living and peace to the dead.

Rue (Ruta graveolens): This plant possesses the power of magic. It is also known as the herb of grace. It is used for blessing, releasing and banishing evil spirits or thoughts.

Sage (Salivia apiana): Sage is used to cleanse objects, places, people and animals. Its aroma has very calming properties.

Sweet Grass (Hierochloe odorata): Sweet grass is also burnt as a purifier, similar to sage. It is lighter than sage and often burnt after burning sage. It encourages positive vibrations to enter the area or room.

Sweet Marjoram (Origanum majorana): Sweet marjoram gives a feeling of comfort in cases of grief and loneliness, since it has a warming effect on the emotions. The Greeks used wild marjoram as a funeral herb and it was planted on graves to bring spiritual peace to the departed.

Thyme (Thymus vulgaris): Thyme is associated with strength and courage.

Yarrow (Achillea millefolium): Yarrow heals wounds on the physical, mental and spiritual level.

Frances Fitzgerald Cleveland has extensive experience in the realms of health and behavior as it relates to both animals and humans. She obtained certification from the Institute of Dynamic Aromatherapy and the International School of Animal Aromatics. Frances studied in England with Caroline Ingraham, the pioneer of Animal Aromatics. Frances is an apprentice of Rosemary Gladstar, world renowned author, herbalist and teacher, and has completed the intensive Apprenticeship Program and the Science and Art of Herbalism Program in the didactic, therapeutic, laboratory and fieldwork in herbalism. She is also a graduate from the University of Connecticut receiving a BA in Journalism and Environmental Science.

Frances recently trained zookeepers in the use of essential oils on animals. Her groundbreaking Animal Aromatherapy work at The Denver Zoo with the Orangutans, Gorillas and Black Crested Macaques was covered in the Denver Post and L.A. Times. Frances' work has also been written about by the Rocky Mountain News, Associated Press, The German Press and a featured guest on Animal Radio.

FrogWorks, Inc. Natural Healing with Plants and Essential Oils for You and Your Animals
Littleton, Colorado
877-973-8848
www.ffrogworks.com
frogworks@att.net

21

When to Get Another Dog
with Jennifer Kachnic, CCMT, CRP

How can I best honor my passing dog?

Should I get the same type of dog?

If you are like most people, you will eventually decide to get another dog after yours has died. This is a personal decision and one that should be made very carefully. The entire family should be involved in deciding the best time to commit to a new relationship. The time frame for this is different for everyone. Bringing a new dog home to the family before everyone is ready can hurt someone by implying that the dog's death is insignificant.

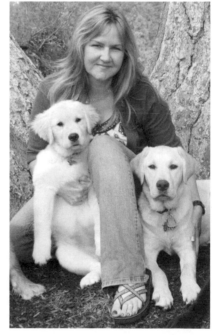

You may feel that you loved your passing dog so much that you can't bear the thought of bringing another dog into your life and going through the loss again. Give yourself time. Try not to rush into making a decision until you have sorted out your feelings and grieved.

Well-meaning friends and family may encourage you to adopt another dog before you are ready. Resist this. When you see a new pair of yearning eyes looking into yours, you will know when you are ready.

During your time of grief, remember to pay attention to the other animals in the home. They also will be affected by the loss of your senior, as well as by your own grief and stress. They may react in various ways, including exhibiting personality or behavioral changes. This is usually temporary. If you have another dog that is suffering from the loss of his senior friend, try to keep his routine as normal as possible and lavish him with attention at this time.

My experience has shown me that one of the greatest legacies you can give your passing dog is to provide your love and compassion to another dog that so desperately needs it. Some people eventually find comfort in going to a local animal shelter and adopting a homeless senior dog. This should be done with some care. Often, people feel that adopting another dog of the same breed and coloring as the dog that has passed will help them deal with their grief. This is usually a mistake. The second dog is not the first dog, and it is unfair to expect him to be. By choosing another dog that is physically different from your passing dog, you will learn to love and appreciate his unique qualities.

If you are not quite sure you are ready for another dog in your life, try fostering an animal through a local animal rescue group. You will not only provide housing and love to a homeless dog while he is waiting for a permanent home, you will be able to test your own readiness without a long-term commitment.

Every dog, especially a senior animal, has so much to offer and will surely enhance and bring joy to your life. If you feel you have grieved and your heart is telling you to open yourself up to another relationship, you are probably ready. For some, there is no better medicine for a hurting heart than the love of another dog, while for others, the best medicine is time.

Jennifer Kachnic has spent her life working and volunteering in animal welfare including fostering hundreds of dogs for local shelters through the years. She is a Certified Therapy Dog Handler for the American Humane Society, Certified Animal Reiki Practitioner and a Certified Canine Massage Therapist. She has been a regular contributor to a variety of pet magazines including Animal Wellness, Mile High Dog Magazine *and* Bark.

As President of The Grey Muzzle Organization, she leads volunteers around the country working to provide grants to animal shelters and rescues nationwide for senior dog programs.

SeniorDogBooks.com
PO Box 3331, Littleton, CO 80161
303-324-3911
Jenny@SeniorDogBooks.com

Facebook: Jennifer.Kachnic
Twitter: SeniorDogBooks
Blog: GreyMuzzle.org/Blog

My Favorite Resource:

ARGUS INSTITUTE

Veterinary Teaching Hospital
Colorado State University

The Argus Institute is a specialized service offering client support within the CSU Veterinary Teaching Hospital. Founded in 1984, our unique program is one of the longest standing, most comprehensive programs of its kind. Our clinical counselors offer support to people who are facing difficult decisions regarding their pet's health and help them manage the challenges of caring for a sick animal.

The Argus Institute provides the following resources:
Advocate for You and Your Pet's Needs

- Fostering the partnership with you and your veterinary care team
- Facilitating decision-making
- Providing updates during surgery and high-risk procedures
- Navigating financial situations
- Assisting during crises
- Pet Hospice Program

Support for Individuals and Families

- Quality-of-life assessment
- Euthanasia decision-making
- Support during euthanasia
- Parent-child discussions
- Grief counseling
- On-line support and resources
- Quality of life assessment tools
- Should I get another pet?

Argus Institute Veterinary Teaching Hospital
Colorado State University
www.ArgusInstitute.colostate.edu
970-297-1242
Argus@colostate.edu

Senior Dog Books
  www.SeniorDogBooks.com

22

Strategies to Cope with Caregiver Suffering with Doug Koktavy

Why do I feel so guilty?

What is my dog trying to teach me at this time?

I used to think grieving was something that began after a loved one passed. So when my nine-year-old Labrador retriever Beezer was diagnosed with kidney disease, it never occurred to me to seek out emotional help for myself during his illness. I could have used it. Beezer was dying, but I was drowning in fear and guilt—fear of what lay ahead when the illness worsened and guilt about my possible neglect in caring for him. Only later did I learn my condition had a name: *anticipatory grief.*

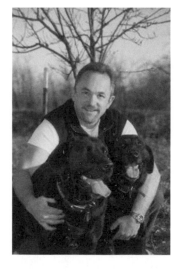

Anticipatory grief: The normal mourning that occurs when a patient or family is expecting a death. Anticipatory grief has many of the same symptoms as those experienced after a death has occurred. It includes all of the thinking, feeling, cultural and social reactions to an expected death that are felt by the patient and family.

People can go through anticipatory grief when pets are dying as well. Today, we are just beginning to understand the scope of the malady related to our own companion animals. Whether it is a person or a pet who is *dying*, symptoms for family members, loved ones and caregivers can include denial, mood swings, anger, frustration, fear, guilt and depression. Anticipatory grief also can lead to physical symptoms, such as weight gain or loss, sleep problems and, in my case, high blood pressure. I came close to being hospitalized for hypertension.

Those of us who are caregivers in particular have a hard time with anticipatory grief. Wrapped up in the day-to-day support of their declining pet, they can feel isolated. Family and friends, busy with their own lives, may deal with the loss when passing actually occurs. This can foster an unsupportive environment during the illness. For better or worse, the caregiver sees the situation in stark reality: a seriously sick animal with growing daily dependence. For the caregiver, the grieving starts now. Recognizing the risk of caregiver anticipatory grief is an important step in developing effective coping strategies.

For me, when Beezer was dying, confusion and difficulty completing tasks were a surprising additional result. As an attorney, running my own practice out of my home, I prized myself on being highly organized, practical and in control. But from the day Beezer was diagnosed, fear and guilt had all the control. It was in; I was out.

Handling Fear and Guilt

Saying that I had a difficult time managing my emotions is an understatement. I was so afraid of losing him, yet over the months that followed, no matter how hard I tried—strict diets, at-home IV treatments, vet visits— I couldn't keep the disease from claiming my pet. Looking back, so much of that journey was consumed by fear. I felt immense fear over what was to come and fear for what my life would be like after Beezer passed. I also felt guilt over my inability to control the outcome. I was used to getting my way by simply working harder; now I had no weapons that worked.

During the time between his diagnosis and our final goodbye, Beezer became my teacher. He and I came to explore the nature of fear and guilt and together we developed strategies to cope. We even learned how to enjoy each day together. But it didn't come easy.

Through this relationship, I came to see that my two biggest problems were deeply tied to time—the past, present and future. I would second-guess and relive past decisions I made on the dog's behalf, under the various headings of:

"Why didn't I try this before?"
"If only I had _____."

and, my personal favorite:

"It's my fault because _____."

These episodes were my ego talking to me, I know that now; not then. My ego was infecting me with guilt over something that happened earlier. I decided that to feel guilty is nothing more than to live in the past.

Moreover, to live in fear is to always live in the future. When this all started happening, the dogs would watch in silent amazement as I rushed about, obsessing over things that hadn't even happened yet. "How much time do we have together?" "What if _____ happens next week?" "Beezer won't even get to celebrate his tenth birthday…"

The problem with this thinking was that my fixation over the future had caused me to ignore today. The key, I finally realized, was to somehow avoid living in both the past and the future. This was presence. Presence is simply living in the moment. This proved to be easier said than done. Anticipatory grief had me in its clutches.

How do you deal with anticipatory grief? First is to acknowledge that the emotions you are going through are normal and can be alleviated. Everyone handles loss differently. Since there were no books back then on dealing with anticipatory grief when a pet is dying, I created my own strategies using what I knew and was familiar with. You may have others.

The Goal of the Disease and My Personal Meaning

During the months I was caring for Beezer, I had a lot of time to think. I began to think about the goal of a fatal disease. It was the enemy. What did it want? It had to be something. The easy response was, "The disease wants to kill Beezer." It sure seemed like it, but was that really the goal?

I gave this some thought. I knew going in that Beezer would die some-day from something. If so, then what did the fatal disease bring to the table that wasn't there yesterday? It couldn't be death, because I under-stood that if you are born, you die. It is our contract from birth.

My answer was that the disease wanted me to give up today. It's just that simple. The goal of a fatal disease is to get me to give up today. The disease accomplishes that goal through fear and guilt.

Because I was losing my buddy, today should have been so very spe-cial. I should have cherished today as never before. Did I? Of course not. I was too busy living in fear of the future that didn't exist today. A mirage in my mind. That was the goal of the disease: To plant the mirage and convince me to live in the future (or in the past, through guilt).

The Embezzler of Today

Now the sneaky part of the disease is that it couldn't rob me of today. It couldn't take today away from me over my objection. It wasn't that powerful. No, the disease had to trick me into giving up today. I would have this wonderful precious asset, today, in my hands and simply hand it over on a silver platter to the embezzler of today, the disease. I'd forfeit today to the con man, as if to say, "Here, you take today, I don't want it. I can't deal with today." Imagine that.

I realized my fear of the disease was the actual fuel that was being used against me. Devilishly clever, my biggest enemy was not the disease, but me. I was the power source being used to generate the very negative energy destroying my own being and wasting a special day with my beloved dog.

This paradox was glaring. I had thought the growing presence of disease was causing my mounting fear. In fact, just the opposite was occurring. My daily increasing fear was causing the disease to become *more powerful*. Faced with this insight, I decided it was high time to start working for me and the Beez, not against us. I came up with three strategies during these trying days.

Strategy #1: The Daily Appreciation

Talking really helps. Beezer, his sibling Boomer and I would gather on the bed and have a nightly discussion. I called them The B Brothers. Each exchange was different yet the same. I'd start with telling them how much they meant to me and how lucky I was to have them in my life. Sometimes we'd talk about fun times. Sometimes we'd talk about the difficult times. I'd explain the illness and my inability to change the outcome. I'd ask for input on how to spend what time we had left together.

Later, as Beezer's time was drawing near, I told him he had my permission and blessing if he wanted to transition on his own. I didn't want him pushing beyond his time because of my selfish needs of wanting to keep him around. I also realized that Beezer might prefer to pass on his own, out of my presence. Of course, that could mean I might come home one day and find that my buddy had left. I decided we needed to talk about that as well. I didn't want any unfinished business or regret after it was too late to say a bit more.

Above all, we always ended on a positive note by expressing our mutual love and deep appreciation for each other. I'd then immediately turn out the lights. I found these discussions of great comfort and continued them with Boomer after Beezer passed and later with my new Lab, Coral.

Strategy #2: Permanent Time-Out

Ever been stuck in traffic? Three lanes and nobody moving? One day that happened to me. I looked around and was puzzled by what I saw in the other lanes. One person was laying on the horn, mouthing single syllable sentences punctuated by some hand gestures. One car over, another person was quietly singing a song of apparent significance. Both people had the same incoming message: "The traffic is stopped." Yet both attached a completely different meaning to the message. I wondered if I could apply this control of the message to my situation with Beezer as he was dying.

I decided that incoming messages are neutral. That is, an incoming message means nothing until the listener attaches a meaning. Up to then, I'd been attaching fear and guilt as the meaning to every incoming message concerning Beezer. I decided to create different meanings to these incoming messages.

I already knew the past (guilt) and the future (fear) were dangerous places for me. My strategy would be to create new meanings that would keep me present. My safe zone was today. Whatever meaning I attached to the disease had to allow me to remain present. I would starve the disease of fuel because it cannot live in the present.

Here was my thought process: The disease was part of our lives. I couldn't change that. I couldn't pretend the illness wasn't here. I had to deal with it, but I needed a way to relate to the disease on terms I could understand. I decided to give the disease a character.

I found an old plastic kiddie chair. I wrote "Kidney Disease Time-Out Chair" on a piece of paper and glued it to the chair. I placed the chair in a prominent place in my house where I could see it often. I then invited the disease to stay, have a seat, but informed it that there were going to be several rules:

1. The disease could never again speak to me without my permission. The disease could hold up signs like, "Can I scare you today?" but planting words in my head was out.

2. The disease could stay in our lives as long as it wanted, but it was restricted to the permanent time-out chair. Beezer and I were busy enjoying today and would try to make time for the disease later. So just sit tight and we'll get back to you.

3. The disease had to wear pink fuzzy slippers. Nothing on this planet is scary when sitting on a kiddie chair wearing pink fuzzy slippers. You play your games, I'll play mine.

I found the strategy helpful. The fact that the chair was out in the open was especially powerful because it reinforced my ability to control fear on a daily basis. Once, when I felt I was becoming anxious again, I composed myself and announced in a stern voice, "WHO SAID YOU COULD LEAVE THE TIME-OUT CHAIR?" It worked. I giggled and both my dogs smiled.

I now had a new power source. I could control the meaning of incoming messages, and thereby change my thinking. The new, healthier thoughts then resulted in a whole new set of emotional responses. Fear and guilt were gone. I was sad about Beezer's illness, but at the same time, I was OK. My new message was that in life, pain is mandatory but suffering is optional. I did not need to suffer. I was returning to a place of balance, perhaps for the first time in a very long time.

Strategy #3: The Daily Point

Well, Beezer passed on, but he left behind a legacy of wisdom with the first lesson being how to live in the moment. The next year, Boomer was diagnosed with bone cancer along with kidney disease. This time I wasn't going to let anticipatory grief undo me. This time my strategy was to remain present by developing a game. Having played ice hockey all my life and being a sports addict, I relish games where scores are kept and winners and losers are determined. Boomer was my equal when it came to fun and games. Our new game was called the Daily Point. Here's how it worked.

Every day, one single point was up for grabs. Either our team, Boomer and I, would get the point or "Team Fear" (now with a second kiddie chair—for the monsters of kidney disease and bone cancer) would get the point. One point each day. There weren't ties and we never had overtime.

Each morning Boomer and I would discuss how we were going to win today's point. We usually came up with something we'd do together. Nothing else mattered. Even on the bad days, we'd stubbornly refuse to give in to fear for the simple reason that we didn't want to lose today's point. We became experts at enjoying today and never looked further than how to win "the point."

Beware of "Martializing the Illness"

A large part of my emotional crisis was caused by always relying on win-related metaphors to guide me. I collectively refer to these metaphors as the Martialization of Illness. You probably are familiar with the common expression, "She waged a heroic battle against cancer." The gist of the metaphors is that loved ones are engaged in "battles" where the opponent is a "monster" and "arsenals" of drugs are called on during the "campaign." Occasionally in this battle of good vs. bad, a being emerges from the campaign with a "victory." These are the "winners." Hooray for the winners!

The problem is, life isn't like that. What happens to the rest of us who aren't the "winners"? The fact is, if you are born, you will one day die. Under a Martialization theory, we'd all become losers at some point in our lives. But people want to win. We are driven to win. Think of sports metaphors. They too can cause an emotional upheaval because you are being set up to fail. The most famous of which emanate from football coach Vincent Lombardi. During Beezer's illness, I'd silently chastise myself for becoming a loser while invoking Lombardi's "Winners never quit and quitters never win" yet another time.

Don't get me wrong, it's good to be challenged occasionally. But when you rely on these words, believe in them, feel you are a failure if you don't win, that's when the crisis can occur.

The problem lies with the effect of these words, and their meaning, on your emotions. In my case, martializing the illness meant the only acceptable outcome was curing an incurable condition. Every other outcome created fear, guilt and a terrific sense that I was letting my dearest friend down in his hour of need. I had to learn, the hard way, that the words and meanings I attached to events created a whole set of negative emotions as a result.

> *Beware of metaphors that can create false expectations, especially in a caretaker's mind, which can have crushing consequences later on.*

* * *

Of course, each journey is unique to the human and the animal. You should follow your instinct and always do what you think is best. *What worked for me is nothing more than what worked for me.*

I believe that everything happens for a reason and that reason helps me grow. I'm a much better person for the lessons about presence taught by these two black dogs and am so deeply appreciative of our time on earth together. The B Brothers helped me learn to overcome fear and guilt and live with presence and balance. Along the way, I realized the abundance of love I showered on my dogs was the same love I withheld from myself. So I learned to forgive Doug. The fellas deserved my love, but so did I.

In retrospect, I found my journey with my B Brothers was never about the body, it was always about the soul. I believe my Labs were sent to earth to teach me lessons I'd never have learned from any other teacher. Because I was able to open up and listen, our journey with kidney disease and bone cancer was the most remarkable success story. A wonderful paradox that I would have missed if I had let myself be consumed by fear and guilt.

Please be kind to yourself and enjoy today with your pet. You'll treasure this most special time for the rest of your life. I think you'll find the best part of your humanity comes forward when your animal becomes ill and you are powerless to change the outcome. We should all be so fortunate to receive such love at the end of our lives.

Below are the **Top Ten Reasons Not to Feel Guilty** that has been excerpted from *The Legacy of Beezer and Boomer: Lessons on Living and Dying from My Canine Brothers* with the permission of Doug Koktavy and his publisher, B Brothers Press.

BEEZER'S TOP TEN REASONS NOT TO FEEL GUILTY

(Compiled by Beezer the Black Lab from the Bridge and sent back to Earth.)

10. Jeez! If you're born, you die. Think about it Dad.

9. Fear is the real enemy, not kidney disease. Fear is curable. I'm with you right now, just invisible. I'll be waiting at the Bridge when you arrive. Don't be afraid. Trust me.

8. Live with balance. The list of what went "right" with my life is so much bigger than the list of what went "wrong." My body died from kidney disease, but my spirit always soared because of you.

7. What you focus on expands. Honor my earthly life and memory. Does feeling guilty help you remember all our good times, adventures and mutual love?

6. Live with Presence! Don't despair about yesterday. Don't fear tomorrow. Otherwise, you'll miss out on the Gift of Today.

5. Thank you for taking my pain into your heart on that last day. I'm so proud of you for that selfless act.

4. Didn't you always forgive me when I made a mistake? I forgive you for any mistake you made during my illness. You made the best decisions possible with the information available at that time. All I took with me on my final earthly journey was our love. Please accept my forgiveness and release the guilt.

3. Pat yourself on the back in between crying. Your effort to treat me was a supreme act of humanity, love and compassion. Our relationship was never more meaningful than during my illness. Please recognize your character and commitment. I do.

2. Guilt is what you humans do to punish yourself for not being perfect.

1. You didn't have a cure for a fatal disease. My body stopped working because of this fatal disease, not because of something you did or did not do.

Doug Koktavy is the author of the multi-award winning book, The Legacy of Beezer and Boomer: Lessons on Living and Dying from My Canine Brothers, *B Brothers Press, Denver, 2010. In 2012,* Managing Caregiver Suffering: A Step-By-Step Guide For Finding Peace in Change *will be released.*

Visit www.BeezerAndBoomer.com *and sign up for free e-training videos, free e-books, and, as a reader of "The Golden Years," enjoy a 50 percent discount on the Guidebook!*

Contact Doug at www.BeezerAndBoomer.com or through email at: Doug@BeezerAndBoomer.com.

My Favorite Resources:

Pet Loss Support Hotline Cornell University
    607-253-3932

IAMS Pet Loss Support Care Center and Hotline
    888-332-7738

ASPCA Pet Loss Support hotline
    877-474-3310

University of Illinois Grief Hotline
    877-394-CARE

Iowa State University Pet Loss Support Hotline
    888-478-7574

Tufts University Pet Loss Support Hotline
    508-839-7966

Washington State University Pet Loss Partnership
    509-335-5704

Pet Loss Support Websites
www.CopingWithYourLoss.com
www.SelfHealingExpressions.com

Pet Loss On-Line Forum
www.HovForum.IPBHost.com

Pet Loss Counseling Services (Doug Koktavy)
www.BeezerAndBoomer.com
Colorado: 303-306-2339
Toll Free: 888-906-2339

University of Colorado Argus Institute
www.ArgusInstitute.Colo.State.edu

Association of Pet Loss and Bereavement counseling
www.APLB.org

Rainbow Bridge

Just this side of heaven is a place called Rainbow Bridge.

When an animal dies that has been especially close to someone here, that pet goes to Rainbow Bridge.

There are meadows and hills for all of our special friends so they can run and play together.

There is plenty of food, water and sunshine, and our friends are warm and comfortable.

All the animals who had been ill and old are restored to health and vigor; those who were hurt or maimed are made whole and strong again, just as we remember them in our dreams of days and times gone by.

The animals are happy and content, except for one small thing; they each miss someone very special to them, who had to be left behind.

They all run and play together, but the day comes when one suddenly stops and looks into the distance. His bright eyes are intent; His eager body quivers. Suddenly he begins to run from the group, flying over the green grass, his legs carrying him faster and faster.

You have been spotted, and when you and your special friend finally meet, you cling together in joyous reunion, never to be parted again. The happy kisses rain upon your face; your hands again caress the beloved head, and you look once more into the trusting eyes of your pet, so long gone from your life but never absent from your heart.

Then you cross Rainbow Bridge together....

Author unknown

Bibliography

Arnold, Jennifer (ed). Through a Dog's Eyes: NY Random House, 2010.

Bailoni, L and Cerchiaro, I. The Role of Feeding in the Maintenance of Well-Being and Health of Geriatric Dogs. Veterinary Research Communications 29(suppl.2)(2005) 51-55.

Brace C, *Journal of Clinical Oncology* (2010;28:2286-2292).

Cooney, Kathy, DVM , Home to Heaven - www.hometoheaven.net/ebook

Coren, Stanley (ed). How Dogs Think –What the World Looks Like to Them and Why They Act the Way They Do: NY SC Psychological Enterprises, 2004.

Fahey, Jr. GC, Barry KA, Swanson, KS. Age-Related Changes in Nutrient Utilization by Companion Animals. Annual Review of Nutrition. 28 (2008): 425-45.

Furman, C. Sue (ed) Balance your dog canine massage, Ft. Collins, CO: Wolfchase, 2003.

Gaynor JS, Muir WW, Handbook of Veterinary Pain Management, Mosby/Elsevier, 2008.

Gina Stewart, Don Kellie Rainwater: When Your Best Friend Becomes Your Old Friend, 2007.

Goldstein, Martin, DVM The Nature of Animal Healing : Ny Random House 1999.

Gregory L. Tillford & Mary L. Wulff, Herbs for Pets, copyright 2009, pg. 238.

Gregory L. Tillford & Mary L. Wulff, Herbs for Pets, copyright 2009, pg. 239.

Gregory L. Tillford & Mary L. Wulff, Herbs for Pets, copyright 2009, pg. 131.

Harper, EJ. Changing Perspectives on Aging and Energy Requirements: Aging and Digestive Function in Humans, Dogs and Cats. *The Journal of Nutrition.* 128:1998. 2632S-2635S.

Hendrickson, DA, Advanced Wound Care, SVMA Syllabus, 2011.

Jones K, et al, IVAPM Statement: Pain Management for End of Life Care, 2011.

Kil, DY, Voler, BMV, Apanavicius, CJ, Schook, LB, and Swanson, KS. Gene Expression Profiles of Colonic Mucosa in Healthy Young Adult and Senior Dogs. PLoS One. (2010) 5(9).

Knueven DVM, Doug. (ed) The Holistic Health Guide. NJ: TFH Publications, 2008.

LaFlamme, DP. Nutrition for Aging Cats and Dogs and the Importance of Body Condition. Veterinary Clinics of North America, Small Animal Practice. 35 (2005) 713-42.

Lascelles BDX, Supportive Care for the Cancer Patient, Ch. 16 in Small Animal Clinical Oncology,4th Ed. Withrow & Vail, Saunders/Elsevier, 2007, p 291-346.

Manteca, X. Nutrition and Behavior in Senior Dogs. Topics in Companion Animal Medicine.Volume 26 (1):2011. p33-36.

McDonald, M, An ethical decision making framework. (Unpublished Document), University of British Columbia Centre for Applied Ethics, 2002. http://www.ethics.ubc.ca.

Morgan, Diane and Wayne Hunthausen, DVM. The Living Well Guide for Senior Dogs: NJ: TFH Publications, 2008.

Morris, JG and Rogers, QA. Assessment of the Nutritional Adequacy of Pet Foods Through the Life Cycle. *The Journal of Nutrition*, 124: (1994) 2520S-2534S.

Mundt, HC. Nutrition of Old Dogs. *The Journal of Nutrition*. 121 (1991) S41-S42.

National Research Council of the National Academy of Sciences. Your Dog's Nutritional Needs. 2006.

Pet food Industry. Many myths about "senior" dog food formula ingredients, researchers find. Pet Food Industry. April 1, 2011.

Rollin BE, Oncology and Ethics, AVMA Proceedings, 2004.

Rollin BE, Animal Happiness, A Philosophical View, Mental Health and Well Being in Animals, ed. McMillan, F.D., 2005, p235-242.

Roudebush, P, Zicker, SC, Cotman, CW, Milgram, NW, Muggenburg, BA, and Head, E. Nutritional management of brain aging in dogs. JAVMA, 227(5): (2005) 722-28.

Satyaraj E, Immunonutrition, Nestle Purina Nutrition Forum: Changing Paradigms in Nutrition, St. Louis, MO, 2008.

Schoen A.(ed.) Veterinary Acupuncture: Ancient Art to Modern Medicine. St. Louis, MO: Mosby Inc 2001.

Smith, Penelope (ed). When Animal Speak: NY Atria, 2009.

Stella JL, Lord LK, Buffington CA, Sickness behaviors in response to unusual external events in healthy cats and cats with feline interstitial cystitis, JAVMA, Vol. 238, No.1, 2011, p. 67-73.

Temel, J.S., Early Palliative Care for Patients with Metastatic Non–Small-Cell Lung Cancer. *New England Journal of Medicine*, 363:8, 8-19-2010, p733-742.

Twedt D, Chronic Vomiting: a practical clinical approach, SVMA Syllalbus, 2011.

Villalobos A, Kaplan L, Canine and Feline Geriatric Oncology: Honoring the Human-Animal Bond, Blackwell Publishing (Wiley-Blackwell), Hoboken, NY, 2007.

Villalobos A. "Pawspice" an End of Life Care Program for Terminal Patients, Ch. 16b, Withrow, McEwen & Vail, Small Animal Clinical Oncology, 4th Ed., W.B. Saunders, Philadelphia PA, 2007.

Voith VL, Attachment of People to Companion Animals, VCNA, Vol. 15, No. 2, The Human-Companion Animal Bond, March 1985, W.B. Saunders Company, Philadelphia PA, 1985.

Wynn S, Marsden S. Manual of Natural Veterinary Medicine: Science and Tradition. St. Louis, MO: Mosby Inc 2003.

Yeates, JW, Main DCJ, The ethics of influencing clients, Views: Commentary, JAVMA, Vol. 237, No. 3, August 1, 2010, p 263-267.

About Jennifer Kachnic

Jennifer Kachnic has spent her life working and volunteering in animal welfare including fostering hundreds of dogs for local shelters through the years. She is a Certified Therapy Dog Handler for the American Humane Society, Certified Animal Reiki Practitioner and a Certified Canine Massage Therapist. She has been a regular contributor to a variety of pet magazines including 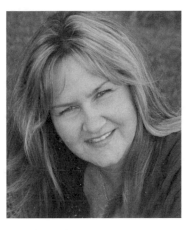 *Animal Wellness, Mile High Dog Magazine* and *Bark.*

As President of The Grey Muzzle Organization, she leads volunteers around the country working to provide grants to animal shelters and rescues nationwide for senior dog programs.

Jennifer also owns and operates a commercial construction company in Denver.

For more information:

SeniorDogBooks.com
PO Box 3331
Littleton, CO 80161
303-324-3911
Jenny@SeniorDogBooks.com

Facebook: Jennifer.Kachnic
Twitter: SeniorDogBooks
Blog: GreyMuzzle.org/Blog